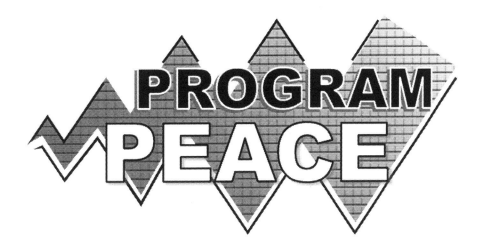

FITNESS MANUAL & JOURNAL

JARED E. RESER PH.D.

Program Peace Fitness Manual and Journal

Jared Edward Reser

ISBN: 9781796239782

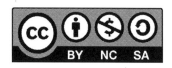

Program Peace: Fitness Manual and Journal

This training manual is intended as a standalone reference and journal. It can also be used as a companion to the Program Peace rehabilitation system found at www.programpeace.com. The information there relates to cutting-edge rehabilitation activities. The information in this book is tried and true, and relates to scientifically accepted diet and exercise knowledge.

Disclaimer

The scientific tables presented in this book were adapted from recent peer-reviewed journal articles. They are meant to promote self-reflection and insight, but not intended as precise medical data. This book is intended to give you the information you need to make healthy lifestyle choices, but is not to be used to diagnose or cure any medical disease or disorder. Improper use of the exercise, diet, massage, and breathing techniques recommended here can lead to self-inflicted harm. Please consult your doctor before starting any new exercise regimen.

About the Author

My name is Dr. Jared Edward Reser. I have been publishing about health, fitness, and brain science, for 15 years. I have two Master's degrees and a Ph.D. in brain and cognitive science from the University of Southern California. I am certified as a personal trainer, health coach, fitness nutrition specialist, functional training specialist, and corrective exercise specialist. I specialize in writing theoretical research articles and place special emphasis on an interdisciplinary approach to integrative biology and cognitive neuroscience. You can find out more about my research at http://www.jaredreser.com.

If Found Please Return To:

My Name: _____

Email: _____

Phone Number: _____

My Fitness Goals:

_____

_____

_____

_____

_____

_____

_____

_____

_____

_____

_____

_____

_____

_____

Table of Contents

Program Peace: Fitness Manual and Journal iii

Preface vii

Introduction viii

Should You See a Doctor Before Starting an Exercise Routine? 1

Metabolism, Exercise, and Weight Loss 2

Calculate Your Resting Metabolic Rate (RMR) 3

Calculate Total Daily Energy Expenditure (TDEE) 4

Calculate Your Daily Fat Needs 5

Calculate Your Daily Protein Needs 6

Carbs, Fiber, Sodium, Sugar, and Water Needs 7

Diet and Nutrition 8

Calculate Your BMI 10

Calculate Your Body Weight Targets 12

Metabolic Measures Progress Chart 15

How Intense Should My Cardio Be? 16

Body Measurements Progress Chart 17

Understanding Your Waist and Hip Circumference 18

Skin Fold Measures 19

Exercise Measures Progress Chart 20

Medical Health Records 21

Cardiovascular Measurements Progress Chart 22

Calculate Your Ideal Exercising Heart Rate 25

Assess Your Balance 26

Mc Gill's Torso Test 27

Flexibility Assessments 28

Optimal Posture 30

Weight Lifting and Resistance Training 31

Reducing Strain and Dormant Muscle. 32

Breathing Exercises. 33

Self-Massage 34

Locations of Muscle Tension 35

List of Exercises. 36

Tips of Staying Active 38

How I feel Before and After 39

Personal Commitment Contract 40

　　　Weekly Excercise Tracker 41

Calendar of Goals and Achievements. 44

　　　Daily Fitness Tracker 47

Preface

Exercise is a potent force for empowerment, healing, and improved health. Exercise produces a range of biological benefits that accumulate over the lifespan. When performed on a regular basis, it decreases blood pressure and lowers resting heart rate. It has been shown to significantly improve anxiety, depression, and a range of other mental health issues. It raises mood, increases social dominance, and acts as a natural painkiller and stress reducer. A range of scientific and medical studies have shown that the benefits include:

Health Benefits of Regular Physical Exercise

- Increased heart strength & capacity
- Increased muscle strength & size
- Increased fluid intelligence
- Improved brain health
- Increased self-esteem & confidence
- Improved sleep quality
- Suppressed appetite
- More efficient fat burning
- Reduced symptoms of depression
- Better cognitive function
- Lower risk of early death
- Lower risk of coronary artery disease
- Lower risk of stroke
- Lower risk of high blood pressure
- Lower risk of high cholesterol
- Lower risk of type 2 diabetes
- Lower risk of metabolic syndrome
- Lower risk of certain forms of cancer
- Weight loss & improved fitness
- Prevention of falls
- Increased bone density
- Increased heart efficiency
- Increased capillary density
- Enhanced lactic acid removal

Most people avoid vigorous exercise because they find it stressful. However, the stress that results from intensive exercise is positive and actually reduces the effects of other, more negative forms of stress. After a workout, you feel happier and calmer due to the release of serotonin, endorphins, and BDNF. These brain chemicals make you feel confident, elated, and accentuate brain cell growth, respectively.

Let's consider endorphin release. Beta-Endorphin is a neurohormone that is released into the bloodstream from the brain's pituitary gland after physical exertion. Endorphins attach themselves to specific receptor sites in the brain that increase our perception of well-being and euphoria. This helps people cope with the effects of mild to severe exertion, and is the way that the body rewards you for exercise. Endorphins also suppress appetite, increase immune activity, aid memory and learning, and decrease sleep disturbances. Even a short jog will give you a significant fraction of a "runner's high." This afterglow of pleasure achieved day after day will program you to be happier, and will motivate you to keep exercising.

Introduction

Research has shown that the exercise your body received as a child plays a tremendous role in your physique and health later in life. The extent of muscle development and fat deposition at puberty is also a major determinant of body type as an adult, but it doesn't stop there. Every time you engage in vigorous activity or eat a healthy meal, you make innumerable positive changes, on a molecular level, to billions of cells throughout your body. Yesterday, today, and tomorrow, you program who you will be in the years and decades to come. This book will guide you on a tour through the most important concepts in exercise and fitness science so that you can totally reprogram yourself, now and for the future.

There are several tables in this book where you can record specific measures. Each table has multiple columns for you to jot down recordings from different dates. The first column gives the name of the measure and its units in parentheses. The arrow after the unit indicates whether you want this measure to increase or decrease. The pages that follow explain how to go about raising and lowering these attributes. It should be both fun and rewarding to watch your personal statistics improve over time.

Date	01 / 03 /XX	02 / 01 / XX	03 / 04 / XX	/ /	/ /
Measure 1 (units) ↑	32.05	36.21	41.67		
Measure 2 (units) ↓	21.97	17.34	13.64		

If you find yourself uninterested in certain pages, gloss over them. If you don't have the body fat scale, or electronic fitness tracker to attain certain measures, skip them. There are many different forms of information in this 50 page manual, and hopefully enough for you to find value in it. Your 90 fitness worksheets for your 90 day fitness challenge start on page 50.

The U.S. Department of Health and Human Services recommends at least 150 minutes of moderate aerobic activity, or 75 minutes of vigorous aerobic activity per week. They also recommend strength training at least twice per week. This book will provide you with the established scientific knowledge you need to meet these goals in a healthful, informed, sustainable way.

You will also be guided to record a chronological history of meaningful health-monitoring data. Do you know your personal metabolic rate? Are you aware of how many grams of fat and protein you should be eating per day? How about calories? Do you know your BMI, lean body weight, or waist-to-hip ratio? Read on and you will! By reading the text and filling in the blanks you will make significant progress in your journey to improved health and fitness.

Should You See a Doctor Before Starting an Exercise Routine?

If you have been diagnosed with a metabolic or cardiovascular disease, you should consult a physician before beginning an exercise routine. If you have 2 or more of the following risk factors, you might also want to consider consulting a physician. This book is not intended as a medical guide. Please report any medical symptoms to a medical doctor.

Disease Risk Factors that Affect Exercise Risk	
Family History	Heart attack, or sudden death before 55 in father, or 65 in mother
Cigarette Smoking	Current smoker or quit within the last six months
Sedentary Lifestyle	Does not participate in at least 30 minutes of moderate-intensity exercise at least 3 days per week
Obesity	Body mass index > 30, or waist girth > 40 inches for men, and > 35 inches for women
Hypertension	Systolic blood pressure > 140 Diastolic blood pressure > 90
Dyslipidemia	LDL > 130 HDL < 40 Total cholesterol > 200
Prediabetes	Fasting plasma glucose > 100

Metabolism, Exercise, and Weight Loss

To maintain a healthy weight, it is important to balance calories in (eating) with calories out (exercise). A positive calorie balance will result in weight gain, and a negative calorie balance will result in weight loss. Because each pound of fat in the body constitutes 3,500 calories, you must reduce your calorie balance by 3,500 calories in order to lose a pound of fat.

> Energy balance = Calories Consumed – Calories Expended

To lose a pound a week you could create a daily 500-calorie deficit by: 1) eating 500 fewer calories per day, 2) burning 500 more calories per day, or 3) eating 250 calories less and exercising 250 calories more. If you can keep any one of these three options up for seven days, then you can create a 3,500 (7 x 500) calorie deficit in a week. This amounts to a full pound of weight loss. Most experts recommend losing between a half-a-pound and two pounds per week. Anything over two pounds lost in a week is considered risky and unsustainable. Remember, only consistent lifestyle changes translate into long-term fitness.

Each pound of fat in your body takes up about as much space as a pint glass or about four sticks of butter. This is about the size of a 450-gram cube with a length of 3.1 inches on each side. So for each pound of fat you lose, your body's volume will decrease by that amount. Five pounds of fat takes up the same space as an American football. So if you are 20 pounds overweight, you have an extra four footballs of fat hanging off your body. Let's burn them off.

Metabolism is the sum of chemical reactions that burn energy within an organism. It literally involves the burning, or combustion, of the food you eat and takes place inside of every one of your body's cells. This literal burning process is part of what makes you warm blooded. To increase your metabolism, you must increase the number of calories that your body burns throughout the day. Our goal is to add lean tissue, and in doing so elevate our resting metabolic rate. As we add lean muscle to our body, that muscle necessitates extra calories to survive. We want enough lean muscle on our bodies that it burns away fat and keeps it from coming back. An additional pound of lean muscle at rest will add an additional 20 to 30 calories to your daily metabolic output. 15 pounds of new muscle will equal around 375 calories per day of added metabolism, and may be enough to ensure a healthy weight. Make it your goal to put on additional muscle mass for this reason.

To really understand your body's metabolism, augment it, and take full advantage of it, let's calculate an estimate for it based on your height, weight, age, and activity level. This will tell you how many calories you can consume each day. It will also give you a baseline to which you add exercise and subtract unneeded calories from. We'll do this on the next page.

Calculate Your Resting Metabolic Rate (RMR)

Here we will use the Mifflin-St. Jeor equation to estimate your resting metabolic rate (RMR). This is the amount of energy your body needs to rest in a reclined position for a full day.

Before you plug your variables into the equation, let's perform the metric conversions in case you measured in pounds and inches. Your weight must be in kilograms, and your height must be in centimeters.

Weight in pounds _____ x .4536 = Weight in kilograms _____

Height in inches _____ x 2.54 = Height in centimeters _____

Men: 9.99 x weight (kg) + 6.25 x height (cm) – 4.92 x age (years) +5 = _____

Women: 9.99 x weight (kg) + 6.25 x height (cm) – 4.92 x age (years) -161 = _____

The number you just calculated will give you a good estimate of the calories that you need to consume just to lie down all day (to calculate this number using a different method, try the Harris-Benedict formula, which can easily be found online). Your RMR is not equal to your daily caloric intake because that must include any physical activity or exercise that you engage in. That is called "total daily energy expenditure," and is calculated on the next page.

Use this chart to keep track of your resting metabolic rate over time.

Date	/ /	/ /	/ /	/ /	/ /	/ /
Resting Metabolic Rate ↑						
Total Daily Energy Expenditure ↑						

Calculate Total Daily Energy Expenditure (TDEE)

In this worksheet, we will use the resting metabolic rate calculated on the last page and multiply it by a number that best describes your level of daily activity. Choose the multiplier from the list below that best describes the intensity of your daily tasks, work environment, and exercise activity.

1.30 Very light activity: Sitting most of the day, talking, little walking, no real exercise.

1.40 Light activity: Slightly below average activity. Some walking, sitting, no real exercise.

1.50 Light to moderate activity: Normal walking, moderate activity, little exercise.

1.60 Moderate activity: Walking and some daily exercise such as jogging or weight lifting.

1.70 Active: Active job, or athletic person engaging in 1-2 hours of exercise per day.

1.80 Heavy activity: Heavy manual labor, or athlete, or 2-4 hours of intense training per day.

_____ X _____ = _____

Resting Metabolic Rate   Chosen Multiplier   Total Daily Energy Expenditure (TDEE)

The number you just calculated is an estimate of the total metabolic energy you expend in 24 hours. This is referred to as total daily energy expenditure, or TDEE. You can use this number to give you an idea of how many calories you need to consume daily to maintain your present weight. Keep in mind that eating more than this will result in weight gain. This is the number that you must alter if you want to lose weight. I want to encourage you to use the dietary journal found later in this book to keep track of all the food you consume over the course of the day. Measuring the total calories consumed and comparing this to your metabolic rate should provide you with some insight into best eating habits. In the next worksheet, we will use your TDEE to calculate your daily fat requirements.

Enter the number that you just calculated for TDEE into the chart on the previous page to keep track of your total daily energy expenditure over time.

Calculate Your Daily Fat Needs

Around 20 to 30% of your calories should come from healthy, unsaturated fats. If you are on a 2,000-calorie-per-day diet then at least 400 calories should be coming from fats. How many grams does that equal? Well, since fats have 9 calories per gram, we can divide 400 by 9 to get 40 grams. Most people require somewhere between 40 and 80 grams of fat each day.

Calculate your daily fat needs:

_____   x   0.25   =   _____   / 9 =   _____

TDEE   Fat factor   Fat calories per day   Grams of fat per day

Some fats are vitally necessary and others are very unhealthy. Remember to choose liquid oils and avoid solid fats. Oils are fats that contain monounsaturated and polyunsaturated fats and are liquid at room temperature. Good sources of these healthy fats include vegetable oils, avocados, nuts, seeds, cheese, eggs, olives and fatty fish.

Avoid saturated fats, which are fats that are solid at room temperature. Saturated fats are commonly found in butter, margarine, ice cream, lard, tallow, whole milk, cream, and fatty meats.

Make an effort to completely avoid trans fats (also known as hydrogenated fats, or partially hydrogenated oils) because they contribute even more than saturated fats to cholesterol buildup and clogging blood vessels. You will want to check nutrition facts labels for trans fats because your recommended daily allowance is zero grams. Trans fats are common in fried fast food, doughnuts, biscuits, cakes, pies, cookies and other fatty snack foods.

Calculate Your Daily Protein Needs

How much protein should you be eating daily? The average person needs between .4 and .8 grams of protein per pound of body weight per day. A sedentary individual should eat between 40 and 90 grams of protein per day. An athlete should intake between 100 and 200 grams of protein every day. To find your optimal intake, use the following table to choose a protein factor to multiply by your body weight in the equation below.

Grams of Protein Needed Per Pound of Body Weight	
Activity Level	**Protein Factor**
Sedentary	.4 grams
Low Level Exercise	.5 grams
Moderate Exercise	.6 grams
Endurance Training	.7 grams
Weight Training	.8 grams

Calculate your daily protein needs:

_____ x _____ = _____

Body weight (lbs.)   Protein factor   Grams per day

Increasing your daily protein intake has benefits. Protein takes more energy to burn than fats and sugars, meaning that increasing the protein in your diet can help boost your metabolism. Also, protein is the macronutrient that is the most difficult to convert into fat. High-protein diets have been shown to be more filling than other types of diets, which can reduce your urge to eat. Consider eating extra protein before and directly after exercise to help in the synthesis and repair of muscle proteins.

Carbs, Fiber, Sodium, Sugar, and Water Needs

You can use the information below to get a good sense of what your daily nutritional targets or ranges should be. However, the following guidelines are not corrected for weight, size, metabolic or disease factors. They are offered here as approximate values. I recommend doing further research and consulting with a registered dietician or medical doctor. Once you get a sense for what your daily target should be, record it below. Then, keep track of your intake day-by-day using your Daily Fitness Journal at the end of this book.

Carbs: Dietary guidelines recommend that carbohydrates provide 45 to 65 percent of your daily calorie intake. On a 2,000 calorie per day diet, you should aim for about 225 to 325 grams of carbs per day. If you need to lose weight you will get much faster results by eating 120 to 200 grams per day. Knowing this, consider a reasonable carb target between 120 and 600 grams.

Carb Target: _____

Fiber: According to the American Heart Association adults on a 2,000 calorie diet should eat around 25 grams of fiber per day. Even higher fiber intakes may reduce chronic disease risk. Large individuals with high metabolisms should consider eating up to 40 grams per day. Consider a daily fiber target for yourself somewhere between 20 and 100 grams.

Fiber Target: _____

Sodium: The American Heart Association recommends no more than 2,300 milligrams (mg) of sodium per day, and advises moving toward no more than 1,500 mg per day for most adults. Unfortunately, Americans consume more than 3,400 milligrams of sodium each day on average. Consider a daily sodium target for yourself between 1,200 and 2,500 milligrams.

Sodium Target: _____

Sugar: The American Heart Association recommends 150 calories (37.5 grams or 9 teaspoons) of sugar per day for men, and 100 calories (25 grams or 6 teaspoons) per day for women. On average, Americans eat more than 300 sugar calories daily. Remember that there is no need for added sugars in the diet, the sugars already available in whole foods are more than sufficient. The less sugar you eat, the healthier you will be. Consider a daily target between 100 and 250.

Sugar Target: _____

Water: Most health authorities recommend that people drink between six and eight 8-ounce glasses of water per day. This amounts to 1.5-2 liters or around half a gallon daily to prevent any form of dehydration. What is your water target?

Water Target: _____

Diet and Nutrition

Use the table below to get a general sense of where your calories should be coming from and how to balance your meals. The information is adapted from highly reliable sources, including the US Nutrition Board, and is promoted on the basis of scientific studies. Check the website for U.S. food recommendations at www.myplate.gov and the website of the American Dietetic Association at www.eatright.org. For individualized dietary advice, see a registered dietician.

USDA ChooseMyPlate.org: Recommended Daily Food Intake For a 2,000 Calorie Diet		
Food Group	Daily Average Over 1 Week	Significance
Grains	6 oz.	Energy and fiber
Whole Grains	4 oz.	
Refined Grains	2 oz.	
Vegetables	3 cups	Potassium, magnesium, fiber, vitamins and minerals
Dark Green Vegetables	.5 cups	
Red / Orange Vegetables	1 cup	
Starchy Vegetables	1 cup	
Beans and Peas	.25 cups	
Other Vegetables	.25 cups	
Fruits	3 cups	Potassium, magnesium, fiber, vitamins, and minerals
Dairy (Low- or Non-Fat)	3 cups	Calcium and protein
Protein Foods (Meat and Eggs)	6 oz.	Protein and magnesium, zinc, vitamin B12
Seafood	9 oz. per week	Protein and magnesium, zinc, vitamin B12, omega 3
Oils	30 grams	Essential fatty acids

Most dietary specialists agree that 25% of the food that you eat should be fruit and 25% should be vegetables. This means that half of every meal should be composed of fruit and vegetables. This equates to 9 servings per day. Eat more veggies and vary them, the darker and more colorful the better. Eat a variety of whole fruits, including fresh, frozen, dried, and canned.

Eat a variety of lean proteins like seafood, lean meat, eggs, beans, peas, nuts, seeds, and soy and whey products. Avoid full-fat dairy but try to eat fat-free dairy daily. Dairy is very nutrient-dense as long as it is fat-free or low-fat. Healthy options can include milk, yogurt, cheese, sour cream, and cottage cheese.

Eat grains (rice, oatmeal, and popcorn), and grain products (bread, cereal, crackers, and pasta). Emphasize whole grains and try to make at least half of your grains whole (e.g., brown rice, quinoa, oats, and whole-grain bread). Whole grains contain the entire kernel and provide enhanced nutritional value.

Make an effort to enjoy your food more, but eat less of it. Eating slowly and mindfully can help. The acceptable macronutrient distribution range is as follows: 45 to 65% of calories should come from carbohydrates, 20 to 35% should come from protein, and 20 to 30% should come from fat. Avoid oversized portions and concentrate on healthy, nutrient-dense foods.

Understanding the concept of nutrient density is important. Foods with added sugar have empty calories and low nutrient density. Nutrient density is the opposite of energy density, also known as "empty calorie" food. Nutrient-dense foods allow you to meet nutrient needs within calorie limits. Take a look at the nutrition facts for two cereals below. Both have a serving size of one cup. One cereal has more calories, more calories from fat, more fat, and more sodium, but less potassium and protein. Which of these two cereals has the higher nutrient density?

Popular Low Sugar Cereal: serving size 1 cup	
Calories	100
Calories from Fat	15
Total Fat	2 g
Sodium	140 mg
Potassium	180 mg
Carbohydrates	20 g
Protein	3 g

Popular High Sugar Cereal: serving size 1 cup	
Calories	173
Calories from Fat	36
Total Fat	4 g
Sodium	293 mg
Potassium	67 mg
Carbohydrates	33 g
Protein	1.3g

Calculate Your BMI

Here we will use the standard Body Mass Index (BMI) equation to estimate your BMI. BMI is a measure of body fat based on height and weight. This number is used by doctors to judge your risk of weight-related health problems. Keep in mind that BMI usually overestimates overfat (overweight) for muscular people and underestimates it for non-muscular people.

Before you plug your variables into the equation, let's perform the metric conversions if necessary. Your weight must be in kilograms, and your height must be in centimeters.

Weight in pounds _____   x .454 = Weight in kilograms _____

Height in inches   _____   x 2.54 = Height in centimeters _____

Height in centimeters _____   / 100 = Height in meters _____

Now, to calculate BMI, you want to square your height in meters (meaning multiply it by itself). Then, take your weight in kilograms and divide it by the number you just got by squaring your height.

BMI = weight (kg) / height (m) ^{2} = _____

Obesity reduces life expectancy by ten to twenty years and increases a number of disease risks. Find your BMI category from the tables on the next page to see your category and disease risks. More than two-thirds of Americans are overweight or obese. So, if your BMI is high, you are not alone, but there is a lot you can do about it, starting today.

BMI Categories	BMI (kg/m^2)	
	from	to
Very severely underweight		15
Severely underweight	15	16
Underweight	16	18.5
Normal (healthy weight)	18.5	25
Overweight	25	30
Obese Class I (Moderately obese)	30	35
Obese Class II (Severely obese)	35	40
Obese Class III (Very severely obese)	40	45
Obese Class IV (Morbidly Obese)	45	50
Obese Class V (Super Obese)	50	60
Obese Class VI (Hyper Obese)	60	

Increased Risk of Obesity-related Diseases				
	BMI			
Disease	< 25	25 – 30	30 – 35	>35
Arthritis	1.00	1.56	1.87	2.39
Heart Disease	1.00	1.39	1.86	1.67
Diabetes (type 2)	1.00	2.42	3.35	6.16
Gallstones	1.00	1.97	3.30	5.48
Hypertension	1.00	1.92	2.82	3.77
Stroke	1.00	1.53	1.59	1.75

Calculate Your Body Weight Targets

This worksheet will help you calculate your body weight targets, meaning a healthy goal weight. To do this, you will need your weight and your body fat percentage. Body fat percentage can be obtained from a body fat scale or monitor. Next, you need to choose your target or ideal body fat. Ideally you should select a target body fat that is between 20% and 5% for men, and 25% and 10% for women. 20 -25% is the maximum for health and 5-10% is the minimum for essential fat. Remember, at 15% you will have a flat stomach, at 10% your abs will show, and less than 10% involves different degrees of vascularity and conspicuous musculature. Select your personal ideal body fat percentage by using the norms found in the tables below. Keep in mind that essential fat and severely underweight are not desirable.

Percentage Body Fat Norms	Men	Women
Severely Underweight	0 - 2 %	0 - 10 %
Essential Fat	2 - 5 %	10 - 13%
Athletes	6 - 13%	14 - 20%
Fitness	14 - 17%	21 - 24%
Acceptable	18 - 24%	25 – 31%
Obesity	> 25%	> 32%

The next two tables will provide you with a subjective "rating system" to help you choose an ideal goal body fat.

Male Body Fat % Rating System						
Age	Unsafe	Excellent	Good	Acceptable	Overweight	Unhealthy
19 - 24	<5%	5-10	10-15	16-19	20-23	>23
25 - 29	<6	6-13	13-16	17-19	20 - 24	>24
30 - 34	<7	7-15	15-18	19-22	23- 25	>25
35 - 39	<7	7-16	17-19	20-23	24 -26	>26
40 - 44	<8	8-18	19-21	22-24	25 - 27	>27
45 - 49	<9	9-19	20-22	23-25	26 - 28	>28
50 - 54	<9	9-20	21-23	24-26	27 - 29	>29
55 - 59	<10	10-20	21-24	25-26	27 - 29	>29
60 +	<10	10-20	21-25	26-27	28 - 30	>30%

Female Body Fat % Rating System						
Age	Unsafe	Excellent	Good	Acceptable	Overweight	Unhealthy
19 - 24	<10%	11 - 19	20 - 22	23 - 25	26 - 29	>29
25 - 29	<12	12 - 19	20 - 22	23 - 25	26 - 30	>30
30 - 34	<13	13 - 20	21 - 23	24 - 26	27 - 31	>32
35 - 39	<13	13- 21	22 - 24	25 - 27	28 - 32	>33
40 - 44	<14	14 - 22	23 - 25	26 - 28	29 - 33	>34
45 - 49	<15	15 - 24	25 - 27	28 - 29	30 - 34	>35
50 - 54	<15	15 - 25	26 - 29	30 - 32	33 - 35	>36
55 - 59	<16	16- 26	27 - 30	31 - 33	34 - 36	>37
60 +	<16	16 - 27	28 - 31	31 - 34	35 - 37	>38%

The following calculations will help you fill out the table on the next page. Start by using a body fat scale to find your weight and body fat percentage. Fill these values into the spaces on the next page below (i.e., 210, 23%).

Then, choose your target body fat percentage from the table above and enter it into the appropriate space (i.e., 12%).

Next, calculate your "number of pounds of body fat" by multiplying your body weight by your body fat. Fill this in (i.e., 210 x .23 = 48).

Then calculate your "lean body weight" by subtracting that last number from your body weight. Fill that in (i.e., 210 – 48 = 162).

To get your "target body weight," divide "lean body weight" by the inverse of "target body fat percentage." To get the inverse, just subtract the number from 1.0 (i.e., 162 / .87 = 186). Fill that in.

Take your "target body weight" and multiply by the "target body fat" to get "target pounds of fat." (i.e. 186 x .12 = 22). Fill that in.

To find "target lean body weight" take your "target body weight," and subtract your "target pounds of fat" (i.e., 184 – 22 = 162). This is the ideal weight that you want to see when you get on the scale.

Finally, to find the number of pounds of fat that you must lose to achieve your targets, take the pounds of fat and subtract "target pounds of fat" (i.e., 48 – 22 = 26). You can then multiply that by 3,500 calories if you want to see the total calories that must be burned to reach the target (26 x 3,500 = 91,000). Or, you can divide your "pounds of fat to lose" by 5 to see how many footballs' worth of space you will shed (26 / 5 = 5.2).

Body Mass by the Numbers:

Body Fat % _____   Target Body Fat % _____

Body Weight _____   Target Body Weight _____

Pounds of Fat _____   Target Pounds of Fat _____

Lean Body Weight _____   Target Lean Body Weight _____

Pounds of fat that must be lost to reach target weight _____

Metabolic Measures Progress Chart

Use the tables below to keep track of changes to your metabolic measures over time. Of course, weight can be measured using a scale. BMI, RMR, and TDEE are calculated based on height and weight from the worksheets above. The rest of the measures can be calculated from the previous section ("Calculating Body Weight Targets").

	/ /	/ /	/ /	/ /	/ /	/ /
Weight ↓						
BMI ↓						
RMR ↑						
TDEE ↑						
% Body Fat ↓						
% Lean ↑						
Fat Weight ↓						
Lean Weight ↑						
Target Body Fat						
Target Body Weight						
Target Pure Fat						
Pounds of Fat to Lose						

The following measures are provided by most body fat scales.

	/ /	/ /	/ /	/ /	/ /	/ /
Basal Metabolic Rate ↑						
% Skeletal Muscle ↑						
Body Age ↓						
Visceral Fat ↓						

How Intense Should My Cardio Be?

Take a look at the following table and the characteristics of the three different zones of intensity for cardiovascular exercise. How much time would you say you spend in each zone during a workout?

Intensity Markers	Zone 1	Zone 2	Zone 3
Talk Test	Talking is somewhat comfortable	Talking is somewhat uncomfortable	Talking is very uncomfortable
Exertion on a scale of 1 - 10	3 - 4	5 - 6	7 - 10
Exertion Level	Moderate exercise intensity	Hard exercise intensity	Very hard exercise intensity
Ventilatory Threshold	Below VT1	Between VT1 and VT2	Above VT2
Percentage of cardio exercise that should be spent in this zone	70%	10%	10%

A variety of different studies of both normal people and athletes have shown that results are maximal when about 70% of cardiovascular exercise is performed in Zone 1, 10% in Zone 2, and 10% in Zone 3.

Body Measurements Progress Chart

Use this chart to keep track of your body circumference measurements. You can take these measurements by wrapping a tape measure around the given body part. The tape should be taut, but shouldn't pinch or depress the skin. Alternatively, you can take the measures with a length of string and then measure the string length against a ruler for more accurate readings.

	/ /	/ /	/ /	/ /	/ /
Right Upper Arm ↓					
Left Upper Arm ↓					
Right Forearm ↓					
Left Forearm ↓					
Right Thigh ↓					
Left Thigh ↓					
Right Calf ↓					
Left Calf ↓					
Waist ↓					
Hips ↓					
Hip / Waist Ratio ↓					

	/ /	/ /	/ /	/ /	/ /
Right Upper Arm ↓					
Left Upper Arm ↓					
Right Forearm ↓					
Left Forearm ↓					
Right Thigh ↓					
Left Thigh ↓					
Right Calf ↓					
Left Calf ↓					
Waist ↓					
Hips ↓					
Hip / Waist Ratio ↓					

Understanding Your Waist and Hip Circumference

The relative location of fat deposits on the body influences disease risk. The apple-shaped fat distribution (fat in the abdominal area) carries greater health risks than the pear-shaped kind (fat on the hips and thighs). This is because abdominal body fat is more easily released into the bloodstream. For this reason, a lower waist-to-hip ratio is preferable. Comparing your waist-to-hip ratio can provide a helpful measure of health monitoring information. This ratio is calculated by dividing the waist circumference that you found in the last section by hip circumference. You want this fraction to be small, and it is best if it is less than 1.0.

_____ / _____ = _____

Waist circumference   Hip circumference   Waist-to-Hip Ratio

Waist-to-Hip Ratio Norms				
Gender	Excellent	Good	Average	At Risk
Male	< 0.85	0.85 – 0.89	0.90 – 0.95	> 0.95
Female	< 0.75	0.75 -0.79	0.80 – 0.86	> 0.86

Criteria for Waist Circumference		
	Waist Circumference	
Risk Category	Females	Males
Very Low	< 27 in	< 31 in
Low	27-35	31-39
High	35-43	39-47
Very High	> 43	> 47

Health Risks Associated with Excessive Body Fat and Waist Circumference
impaired cardiac function due to increased workload on the heart; hypertension; stroke; heart disease; high blood pressure; diabetes; deep-vein thrombosis; increased insulin resistance; renal disease; sleep apnea; pulmonary disease; problems receiving anesthesia during surgery; osteoarthritis; degenerative joint disease; gout; endometrial, breast, prostate, colon and other cancers; abnormal plasma lipid and cholesterol levels; gallbladder disease; psychological stress; social stigma; and discrimination.

Skin Fold Measures

Use this chart to keep track of your body skin fold measures. These are taken by measuring folds of body fat using calipers and are used to estimate body fat percentage. Detailed measuring instructions can be found online, or you can have these measures taken professionally. You generally want these numbers to decrease, unless you have a BMI under 20.

Men	/ /	/ /	/ /	/ /	/ /	/ /
Above Knee ↓						
Abdomen ↓						
Chest ↓						
Total (mm)						
Body Fat						

Women	/ /	/ /	/ /	/ /	/ /	/ /
Above Knee ↓						
Supraillium ↓						
Tricep ↓						
Total (mm)						
Body Fat						

Men	/ /	/ /	/ /	/ /	/ /	/ /
Above Knee ↓						
Abdomen ↓						
Chest ↓						
Total (mm)						
Body Fat						

Women	/ /	/ /	/ /	/ /	/ /	/ /
Above Knee ↓						
Supraillium ↓						
Tricep ↓						
Total (mm)						
Body Fat						

Exercise Measures Progress Chart

This table lists some of the most common exercise tests. A quick Internet search will provide the information needed to administer each test. Write down your scores, and have fun keeping track of how they improve as your fitness improves. You can list other measures in the blank spaces below.

	/ /	/ /	/ /	/ /	/ /
Plank (sec) ↑					
Wall Sit (sec) ↑					
Push-Ups / min ↑					
Pull-Ups / min ↑					
Crunches / min ↑					
Squats / min ↑					
1 Rep Max Bench (lbs) ↑					
1 Rep Max Squat (lbs) ↑					
Vertical Jump (inches) ↑					
Long Jump (inches) ↑					
40 Yard Dash (sec) ↓					
300 Yard Shuttle Run (sec) ↓					
T test (sec) ↓					
Pro Agility Test (sec) ↓					
3-Minute Step Test ↓					
Fit Test ↓					
Kneeling Overhead Toss (feet) ↑					

Medical Health Records

Use this chart to keep track of important medical health measures and lab test results. These tests are administered by your healthcare provider. You can list other measures in the blank spaces below.

	/ /	/ /	/ /	/ /	/ /	/ /
Blood Pressure (mmHg) ↓						
Total Cholesterol (mg/dl) ↓						
Triglycerides (mg/dl) ↓						
HDL (mg/dl) ↑						
LDL (mg/dl) ↓						
Fasting Glucose (mg/dl) ↓						
Cortisol ↓						
T4 (ng/dl)						
TSH (uIU/mL)						
Creatine (U/L)						
Estrogen						
Testosterone (ng/dL)						
Sodium (mEq/L)						
Potassium (mEq/L)						
Chloride (mEq/L)						
Calcium (mg/dL)						

Cardiovascular Measurements Progress Chart

Use this chart to keep track of your cardiovascular measures. Heart rate can be assessed using a heart rate monitor or by counting your own pulse over the course of a minute. Blood pressure can be found using a syphgmomanometer, inspiratory volume by using an inspirometer, and heart rate variability and VO2 max can be assessed using a smart watch. These measures are explained in detail on the following pages.

Date	/ /	/ /	/ /	/ /	/ /
Resting Heart Rate (bpm) ↓					
Max Heart Rate (bpm) ↑					
Estimated Max Heart Rate					
Heart Rate Range (bpm) ↑					
Blood Pressure (mmHg) ↓					
Heart Rate Variability ↓					
VO2 Max ↑					
Max Inspiratory Volume (ml) ↑					
VT 1 (bpm) ↑					
VT2 (bpm) ↑					
Breath Hold (sec) ↑					
Breaths / Min. at Rest					
Breaths / Min. During Sleep					

Resting Heart Rate

Resting heart rate is a measure of heart activity expressed in beats per minute. Regular exercise training increases the amount of blood that the heart pumps per stroke. This leads to reductions in heart rate. Because of this, athletes commonly have heart rates under 50 bpm. However, most people with a resting heart rate lower than 50 (bradycardia) or higher than 100 (tachycardia) should consult a medical professional. Otherwise, take note of and record your resting heart rate for future comparisons. To do so, take your heart rate after sitting for 3 minutes on three separate occasions, and take the average of the three measurements.

Classification of Resting Heart Rate	
Bradycardia	< 60
Too Low	0 - 40
Athlete	40 - 60
Normal	60 - 100
Average	72
Tachycardia	>100

Maximum Heart Rate

In general you want your resting heart rate to be low, but you want your maximal heart rate to be high. As we age, our maximal heart rate declines every year. This means that the intensity at which the heart is capable of pumping blood decreases with natural aging. A reliable way to estimate your maximum heart rate is to take 208 and subtract 70% of your age (208 − .7 x AGE). You can enter this number in the table on the previous page. Alternatively, you can find your actual maximum heart rate using your pulse or a smart watch (or the electrodes available on most gym cardio equipment) during high-intensity exercise. Regular exercise will help you maintain a high maximal heart rate.

Heart Rate Range

Heart rate range is found by subtracting resting heart rate from maximum heart rate. Generally the higher your heart rate range, the better. Also, the quicker your heart rate drops after strenuous exercise, the healthier your heart.

Blood Pressure

Blood pressure is a measure of the pressure that circulating blood places on the walls of blood vessels. Excessive pressure is damaging and promotes the accumulation of plaque inside vessels. Blood pressure is usually expressed as a fraction (e.g., 115/78). If the top number is over 120 or the bottom number is over 80, or both, then your blood pressure is likely high to an unhealthy extent. See the table below for more information. Regular exercise and healthy eating promotes lower blood pressure.

Classification of Blood Pressure for Adults		
	Systolic	Diastolic
Normal	< 120	< 80
Prehypertension	120 - 139	80 – 89
Hypertension		
Stage 1	140 – 159	90 – 99
Stage 2	>160	>100

Heart Rate Variability

Heart rate variability (HRV) is a measure of variation in the time interval between heart beats. Low HRV is a sign of a fight-or-flight stress system that is turned up too high. If your HRV values are higher than your comparable age-gender demographic range, this suggests that your biological age is younger than your chronological age. HRV can be measured by a professional or can be estimated by some smart watches or home kits. Regular exercise may be the best way to raise your HRV, stress resilience, and composure.

VO$_2$ Max

VO$_2$ Max is a measure that reflects cardiorespiratory fitness and endurance capacity. It is often taken to be an indicator of athleticism. VO$_2$ Max can be measured by a professional or can be estimated by some smart watches or home kits. Again, the more exercise you perform, the higher you can expect your VO$_2$ Max to climb.

Max Inspiratory Volume

Max inspiratory volume is the maximum amount or volume of air that can be inhaled after a full exhalation. Some professionals see this as a measure of respiratory health. This volume can be increased by regular exercise and breathing exercises that target the diaphragm such as taking full smooth breaths.

Calculate Your Ideal Exercising Heart Rate

This worksheet will help you determine how many beats per minute your heart should be at during cardiovascular exercise. Knowing this will help you adjust your exercise intensity accordingly. First, you will need to determine your maximum heart rate. A fast and reliable way to do this is by using the equation below.

208 – (.7 x AGE) = _____ = Maximum Heart Rate (MHR).

Once you have your max heart rate, then subtract your resting heart rate from this number to obtain your heart rate range. Your resting heart rate can be taken using a heart rate monitor or by counting your pulse while at rest.

Max Heart Rate – Resting Heart Rate = _____ = Heart Rate Range (HRR)

To find your target heart rate range for moderate aerobic exercise, multiply your heart rate range by .5, and then by .7. This will give you two numbers, 50% and 70% of your heart rate reserve. Add your resting heart rate to both of these numbers to get your range of target heart rates.

(HRR x .5) + RHR = _____ = Low range of target heart rate

(HRR x .7) + RHR= _____ = High range of target heart rate

A large proportion of your cardiovascular exercise should be taking place in the zone between these two target heart rates if you intend to exercise moderately.

To find your target heart rate range for vigorous aerobic exercise, multiply your heart rate range by .7, and then by .8. This will give you two numbers, 70% and 80% of your heart rate reserve. Add your resting heart rate to both of these numbers to get your range of target heart rates.

(HRR x .7) + RHR = _____ = Low range of target heart rate

(HRR x .8) + RHR= _____ = High range of target heart rate

A large proportion of your cardiovascular exercise should be taking place in the zone between these two target heart rates if you intend to exercise vigorously.

Assess Your Balance

Sharpened Romberg Balance Test:

This test assesses static balance. Remove your shoes. Stand straight with one foot directly in front of the other. Fold your arms across your chest with each hand touching the opposite shoulder. Close your eyes before you begin and try to retain your balance without moving or taking a step for 60 seconds. Measure your balance time when you right leg is in front, and then take the measure again with the left leg in front.

Right Leg in Front	Left Leg in Front	Difference

60 seconds is a perfect score. Inability to reach 30 seconds indicates inadequate static balance. Keep practicing.

Stork Stand Balance Test:

This test is an alternative way to assess static balance in a modified position. Remove shoes. Place the hands on the hips. Raise one foot off of the ground and bring the bottom of the foot to lightly touch the inside of the stance leg, below the knee. Balance on the ball of the foot, with the heel off the ground. Try to retain balance for 60 seconds

Right Leg on Ground	Left Leg on Ground	Difference

Use this chart to keep track of your balance scores

Date		/ /	/ /	/ /	/ /	/ /
Sharpened Romberg	↑					
Stork Stand	↑					

The ability to maintain these positions without falling or moving the feet for 30 seconds indicates good balance and postural control. More than 50 seconds is excellent and can be approached with practice.

Mc Gill's Torso Test

Mc Gill's Torso Test will provide you with a good understanding of how balanced your lower back and core strength is. You can easily find descriptions for each of the three tests online.

Trunk Flexion Endurance:

Time held: _____

Trunk Extension Endurance:

Time held: _____

Trunk Lateral Endurance:

Right-side held: _____

Left-side held: _____

Flexion : extension ratio: _____/_____ = _____ Should be less than 1.0.

Right-side bridge : left-side bridge ratio: : _____/_____ = _____ Should be no greater than 0.05 from a balanced score of 1.0.

Side bridge (each side) : extension ratio: : _____/_____ = _____ Should be less than 0.75.

Use this chart to keep track of your torso test results over time.

Date		/ /	/ /	/ /	/ /	/ /
Flexion	↑					
Extension	↑					
Lateral	↑	/	/	/	/	/

Flexibility Assessments

The following are standard flexibility assessments for which you can easily find testing instructions online. Pay careful attention to the form and assessment criteria. Flexibility training should be done after a workout when the muscles are more elastic. Remember that warming up is important to increase the range of motion of the muscles.

Thomas Test		
	Normal	Tight
Left Hip		
Notes		
Right Hip		
Notes		

Passive Straight-leg Raise		
	Normal	Tight
Left Hamstring		
Notes		
Right Hamstring		
Notes		

Shoulder Flexion		
	Normal	Tight
Left shoulder		
Notes		
Right shoulder		
Notes		

Shoulder Extension		
	Normal	Tight
Left shoulder		
Notes		
Right shoulder		
Notes		

Internal Rotation		
	Normal	Tight
Left shoulder		
Notes		
Right shoulder		
Notes		

External Rotation		
	Normal	Tight
Left shoulder		
Notes		
Right shoulder		
Notes		

Apley's Scratch Test		
	Normal	Tight
Left reach-under		
Notes		
Left reach-over		
Notes		
Right reach-under		
Notes		
Right reach-over		
Notes		

Some Helpful Yoga Poses for Flexibility, Mobility, and Joint Health

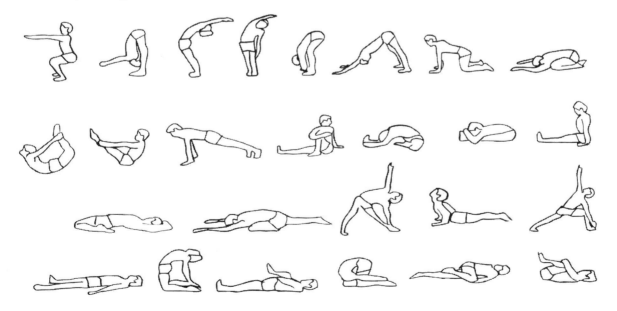

Optimal Posture

Five Steps for Optimal Posture

1) Set your feet straight ahead, and let the rest of your body follow, with no twisting.
2) Tilt your hips backward and contract your gluteus muscles rather than tilting your hips forward, arching your back, and sticking out your butt.
3) Tighten the abdominals and tuck the stomach in slightly by drawing your bellybutton to your spine.
4) Pull your shoulders back and down. Spread your chest and lean your mid-back backwards, instead of shrugging and slumping forwards.
5) Make sure that your head is pulled backwards and your chin is tucked in toward your chest. Next, pull your chin towards your Adam's apple. You don't want your head hanging forward and your jaw jutting out.

Posture Check: Frontal View

- ☐ Left and right sides of the body should be symmetrical
- ☐ Ankles should not be supinated or pronated
- ☐ Feet should be facing forward, and not be inverted or everted
- ☐ Knees should be the same height and orientation with no rotation
- ☐ Hips should be the same height with no shifting, and alignment of the iliac crests
- ☐ The bellybutton, sternum, neck, and pubis should be on the plumb line
- ☐ Shoulders should be equal height, low, and not rotated inwards
- ☐ Arms should be relaxed at the sides with equal distance from arm to torso on each side
- ☐ Hands should be facing the thighs
- ☐ Ears, nose, eyes, and chin should be facing forwards, possibly slightly lifted
- ☐ Spine should be straight, and all vertebrae should be in alignment
- ☐ Shoulder blades should be neither winged nor pronated

Posture Check: Side View

- ☐ Load-bearing joint landmarks should be aligned with the plumb line
- ☐ Knees should be slightly bent
- ☐ The ASIS and PSIS should be at exactly the same height
- ☐ Observe for excessive curving of the spine: thoracic kyphosis, lumbar lordosis, or flat-back position
- ☐ Shoulders should be held back without forward rounding (protraction) of the scapulae
- ☐ The neck should be retracted with the ear in line with the acromion of the shoulder, and the cheek in line with the collar bone.

Weight Lifting and Resistance Training

Effective weight training will create tiny microtears in muscle fibers. When the body heals these tears, the fibers are built back stronger and larger. The healing process takes from 4-6 days for heavily exercised muscle, so to really achieve full recovery you should give yourself at least 4 days of rest. Does this mean that you should only work out once a week? Of course not. Instead, you should exercise different body parts on different days. Many people divide their week into push day, pull day, and leg day. If you want to lift heavy weights more than three times per week, you can divide the week into chest day, back day, ab day, shoulder day, and leg day. Parceling your time out in this way is necessary to avoid overtraining and overuse injuries.

How many repetitions you perform will determine what kind of changes you see in your body. Keep in mind that each of the repetition counts listed below should end in complete muscle contraction failure and an inability to do one more repetition.

Endurance / Conditioning / Toning:

15 to 20 repetitions per set. The twentieth rep should be a struggle. Once you can do 21, its time to up the weights or slow down the repetitions.

Bodybuilding / Hypertrophy / Muscle Size:

8 to 12 repetitions per set.

Strength:

5 to 8 repetitions per set.

Power:

3 to 5 repetitions per set.

Most people want to see an increase in muscle size, and the best way to achieve this is to perform at least three sets with 8 to 12 repetitions. This should be performed with weight that is around 80% of the 1-repetition maximum. Once you can perform more than 12 reps, increase the weight by 5 to 10%. After each set, you should allow up to three minutes of rest for that particular muscle group, meaning that you can exercise other muscle groups during this time.

Each rep should take more than 2 seconds. A good time under tension is 3 seconds per rep (1 for the contraction, and 2 for the decontraction). Some lifters strongly advocate working the negative. This involves decontraction of a muscle as it elongates. An example would be lowering the dumbbell very slowly after a bicep curl, or lowering slowly to the ground after a push-up. The negative decontraction may result in more microtears and thus more growth.

Reducing Strain and Dormant Muscle

Intense exercise and especially weight lifting increase muscle tension. Over time, it will cause discomfort and pain if left untreated. When this happens, it is often referred to as overtraining, overuse, or repetitive strain injury. The smaller muscles that line the spine, shoulders, and hips are particularly susceptible, especially if they stay tight after a workout. If muscle tension is not released, it will cause the muscle to go into dormancy, involving a number of cellular changes that make it hard, weak, and painful. Dormant muscle is stuck in a state of partial contraction. There are reliable ways to prevent and reduce dormant muscle, and they include:

The Use of Light Weights: The heavier the weight, and the fewer the reps (3-8), the more tension you create, and the higher the likelihood of cramping and injury. Less weight and numerous reps (12-50) build strength more slowly, but more safely, and less reversibly.

Massage: Regular full-body massage will increase circulation and reduce muscular restrictions. You want to press firmly into the sore and achy muscle to release it.

Stretching: Stretching or yoga after a workout will keep your muscles limber and supple, and increase their ability to support your body weight against the force of gravity.

Postural Awareness: Exercising with bad posture will make posture worse. Maintaining proper posture throughout the day and being aware of the tendency to hold tension in certain body parts will significantly reduce cumulative strain.

Full-Range Contraction: You want to perform contractions throughout every muscle's full range of motion. The antifrailty protocol below describes how best to do this.

Antifrailty Protocol

1) Locate an area of the body that is stiff and achy when held in an active stretch or contraction. The point where this configuration cracks is likely the most in need of rehabilitation. Hold the achy postural configuration for five to thirty seconds.

2) Hold the general parameters of the posture while varying others. Move the joint dynamically, utilizing its range of motion in every possible vector and flexing into those that seem the stiffest or sorest. Stretch into it right up until it cracks. If it does crack, then freeze and hold that posture for an additional five to fifteen seconds.

3) Allow the area at least fifteen seconds of complete rest before you resume.

Antifrailty will allow you to rehabilitate and strengthen your body's weakest areas. To get the best results, combine it with light weight lifting, yoga, and/or breathing exercises.

Breathing Exercises

Most people breathe neurotically because their respiratory diaphragm is strained and stuck in a state of partial contraction. This causes us to breathe short breaths shallowly and erratically. When the diaphragm is tense in this way, psychological stress is unavoidable. In fact, any traumatized mammal will have a tense diaphragm and breathe shallowly. The following exercises guide you to rehab your diaphragm so that you can breathe easy. These exercises will be uncomfortable at first, but will become more comfortable with time.

Blow on Finger: Purse your lips and blow on your fingertip until you can no longer feel your breath on your finger. Just one full evacuation of the lungs is often enough to kick-start diaphragmatic breathing because the resulting vacuum automatically pulls the diaphragm through its full bottom-end range of motion. Repeat this five times per day.

15 Second Inhale: Set a timer or watch the second hand on a clock, and inhale slowly and smoothly for no less than 15 seconds. This teaches your nervous system that it is safe to breathe slow, deep breaths. As a mammal, this is the most comforting message you can send to your unconscious brain.

Listen to the Smoothness of Your Breath: Cup both hands between your mouth and ear, creating a bridge for the sound of your breath. The breath should be louder, and the discontinuities in your breath should be more apparent. You want to listen for brief cessations or unevenness in the sound. Concentrate on making the breath perfectly smooth and even so that these disturbances disappear. Do not let the rate change. This will iron out the apneic disturbances in your diaphragm's range of motion that influence you to startle.

Perform Paced Breathing: Download a breathing application or breath metronome on your phone or tablet to perform paced breathing. Starting with 4-second inhalations and 6-second exhalations is a great place to start. The app will guide you, telling you when to inhale and when to exhale. Try to inhale and exhale completely with each prolonged breath. The more you use the breath metronome, the more you will program yourself to be able to breathe diaphragmatically without it.

Nasal Breathing: Breathing through the nose narrows the pathway of air and forces your diaphragm to work harder and more evenly. This is why nasal breathing builds strong, steady respiratory function and, once strengthened, makes you a calmer person.

Diaphragmatic Reading Out Loud: Sit down with a good book and begin reading aloud. When you do so, take a slow, full breath in and then read aloud until you have no breath left to exhale. Do this repeatedly for five minutes. You should find that you inhale for somewhere between 5 and 10 seconds, and that you speak/exhale for between 6 and 12 seconds.

Self-Massage

Muscles that feel tender when subjected to deep compression are the muscles you have neglected to provide breaks. They hurt because they never get to rest. Compression gives them that much-needed break and reestablishes blood flow and full regeneration. Often the muscle will feel warm afterwards as fresh blood rushes to neglected areas. You want to perform *ischemic compression*; literally squeezing the blood out of the tissue. Compression creates the cellular events necessary to express the genes necessary to build new blood vessels. Daily massage will bring your muscles back to life.

Compression Protocol

1) Find a muscle that is tender when compressed. Press firmly on the muscle with the tip of the thumb, a knuckle, the heel of the palm, or a tool. You want to squeeze for somewhere between 5 and 30 seconds. The compression of each area should take less than a minute. On most areas of the body, you can apply between 5 and 25 pounds of pressure. Release and then reposition to an adjacent area and repeat.

2) Some practitioners recommend sliding down the length of the muscle. Use deep, firm strokes, moving in the direction of the muscle fibers. Others recommend stroking across the muscle repeatedly, like strumming a guitar string. Either way, you want to pin the skin down and slide over the muscle rather than sliding over the skin.

3) On a scale of 1 to 10, aim for a pain level of 6 or 7. The pain should be right at the edge of tolerable discomfort before you squirm, brace, or breathe shallowly. You want to be breathing long, slow breaths while doing this.

4) Once you release the muscle, try to notice how the bracing in this muscle has diminished and how you feel insecure or exposed now that you are no longer bracing it. Note the automatic tendency to either resume the bracing or breathe shallowly. Continue to breathe deeply while unbracing to force the muscle to reset to a lower level of tone.

5) The next day, the muscle should be completely unbruised but lightly sore to the touch. If it is sore when contracted, that means that you went too hard. The sore-to-the-touch sensation means that you performed the compression properly. The muscle will ache more now when compressed that it did the day before, but after compressing it for a minute this soreness should disappear. After the soreness disappears, wait a few hours for it to come back, and compress it again to the same extent. Repeat this process until the muscle is painless to compress. Depending on the size of the muscle and the severity of the tension, this could take days, weeks, or months.

Locations of Muscle Tension

The charts below are designed for you to use a pen or pencil to mark points of muscle tension on your body. You can mark different forms of tension using the following symbols:

X = Use this to indicate injury or pain that should be treated carefully.

O = Use this to indicate tight, stiff, inflexible muscle that needs to be stretched.

Δ = Use this to indicate muscle that is sore when massaged and needs to be compressed.

□ = Use this to indicate muscle that is achy when contracted, and thus needs antifrailty.

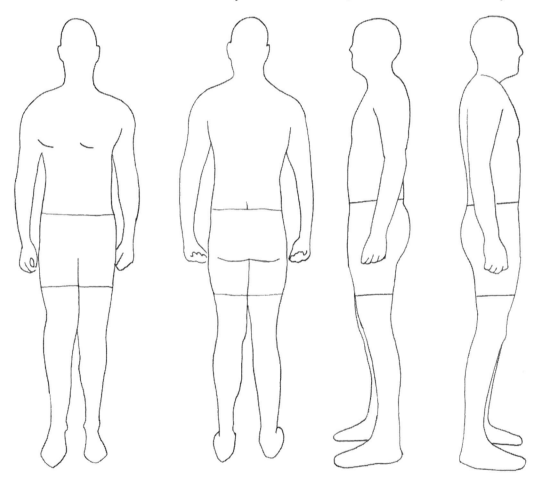

List of Exercises

Need some good exercises to use to fill in the spaces in your training journal? Below you will find some of the best. A quick online search will fill you in on form and function.

Body Weight Exercises & Calisthenics

Bear Crawl, Birddog, Burpees, Butt Kicks, Candle Stick, Carioca, Chain Breakers, Cone Jumps, Corkscrew, Crab Walk, Diagonal Cone Jumps, Donkey Kicks, Fitboard, Flutter Kicks, Forearm Plank, Full Body Bridge, Glidewalking, Glute Bridge, Goodmornings, Head Cradle Hip Hinge, Hexagon Drill, High Knees, High Knees, High Marches, Hip Bridges, Hops/Leaps/Bounds/Depth Jumps, Inch Worms, Incline Plyometric Pushup, Jumping Jacks, Jumping Lunges, Jumps in Place, Kegels, Kettle Bell Swings, Lateral Shuffles, Multidirectional Drill, Cutting Drills, Mountain Climbers, Plank Jacks, Prisoner Rotations, Pronearm Lifts, Roll Foam Roller Down Spine, Russian Twists, Side Plank, Sit Ups With Head Turned to Side, Sitting Knee Tucks, Situp Crunches, Skaters, Sprinters Sit Up, Squat Jacks, Step Ups, Stutter Step, Toe Touch, Walking with Abs Flexed and Bellybutton to Spine

Stretches:

90/90 Stretch, Butterfly Stretch, Calf Stretch, Chest Corner Stretch, Cross-Body Shoulder Stretch, Figure Four Stretch, Frog Stretch, German Hang, Knee-to-Chest Stretch, Lunge with Spinal Twist, Lunging Hip Flexor Stretch, Lying Knee Twist, Lying Pectoral Stretch, Lying Quad Stretch, Piriformis Stretch, Pretzel Stretch, Runner's Stretch, Seated Groin Stretch, Seated Neck Release, Seated Shoulder Squeeze, Seated Trapezius Stretch, Seated Trunk Twist, Side Bend Stretch, Standing Hamstring Stretch, Standing Oblique Stretch, Standing Quad Stretch, Standing Side Stretch, Swan Stretch ,Triceps Stretch

Yoga Poses:

Awkward, Boat, Bow, Box, Bridge, Camel, Caterpillar, Chair, Childs, Cobra, Corpse, Cow, Crescent, Crow, Dolphin, Downward Dog, Eagle, Easy, Fire Log, Firefly, Fish, Forward Fold, Frog, Garland, Gorilla, Half Moon, Handstand, Happy Baby, Head-to-Knee, Headstand, Hero, Pigeon, Locust, Lotus, Lunge, Mountain, Pigeon, Plank, Plow, Pyramid, Rabbit, Shoulder Stand, Side Angle, Sphinx, Splits, Staff, Table, Tree, Triangle, Warrior, Wheel

Cardiovascular and Aerobic Exercises:

Aquarobics, Boxing, Cardio Classes, Cycling, Cross Country, Dancing, Eliptical, Hiking, Jogging, Jumping Jacks, Jumping Rope, Rowing, Running, Skateboarding, Swimming, Stair Climbing, Team Sports, Walking

Sports:

Badminton, Baseball, Basketball, Boxing, Cheerleading, Cricket, Dodgeball, Football, Handball, Hockey, Lacrosse, Martial Arts, Racquetball, Rugby, Soccer, Softball, Skating, Skiing, Tennis, Volleyball, Wrestling

Group Classes:

Body Works, Bootcamp, Cardio Kickboxing, Cross Fit, Dance, Jazzercise, Jiu-Jitsu, Karate, Krav Maga, Muay Thai, Pilates, Salsa Dancing, Spinning, Step Aerobics, Tae Kwon Do, TRX, Turbo Kick, Water Aerobics, Yoga, Zumba

Plyometric Exercises:

Box Jump, Clapping Pushup, Heisman Move, Lateral Jump, One-Leg Box Jump, Pike Jump, Power Skip, Single-Leg Tuck Jump, Speed Skater, Squat Jump, Tuck Jump, Vertical Jump and Reach

Weight Lifting Exercises:

Back Extension, Bench Press, Bent Over Rows, Calf Raise, Chair Dips, Chest Fly, Crunch, Incline Press, Lateral Raise, Leg Curl, Leg Extension, Leg Press, Leg Raise, Lunge, Military Press, Preacher Curl, Pull-down, Pull-up, Push Down, Push Ups, Reverse Flys, Shoulder Press, Shoulder Press, Shoulder Raise , Shoulder Shrugs, Squat, Torso Turns with Barbell, Upright Row, Woodchops and Haybailers, Yates Row, Zottman Curl

Power Lifting Exercises:

Front Raise, Hang Cleans, Jefferson Squat, One Arm Kettle Bell Snatch, Overhand Sumo Dead Lift, Overhead Squat, Power Clean, Power Snatch, Push Jerk, Push Press , Shoulder Press , Split Jerk , Squat Clean, Squat Snatch, Straight Leg Deadlift, Strict Press

Tips for Staying Active

- Walk and stretch at lunch and during other work breaks.
- Avoid escalators, elevators, and other labor-saving devices.
- Have a walk-and-talk meeting rather than sitting at a desk.
- Work while standing, use a standing or hybrid desk, or place your laptop on a bookshelf.
- Pace, stretch, self-massage, or perform breathing exercises while on the phone.
- Walk with your children or spouse and talk about their day.
- Choose the furthest parking spot from your destination.
- Keep headphones, water bottles, and a change of clothes in the car to limit excuses.
- Listen to books on tape while you work out so that you can feel even MORE productive.
- Habits are easy to keep going once you develop them. So being disciplined only gets easier.
- Set up your phone charger on the floor. Bend down slowly, with control, and a long even exhale every time you pick up your phone.
- Remember that exercise decreases physiological stress and increases mental happiness.
- Get your friends and family to exercise with you.
- Self-control is a limited resource, so minimize the amount needed by setting yourself up for success in advance.
- Changing your lifestyle takes time and effort, so start with small, manageable goals.
- Use the pedometer on your smart phone.
- Consider purchasing a fitness tracking watch to record and monitor your calorie count, to stay motivated, and to get daily feedback on your biometrics so that you can learn from them.
- Focus on creating positive, fun, and exciting exercise experiences.
- Think of yourself as getting healthier and stronger every day.
- Make improvements in multiple areas such as stretching, drinking more water, eating healthier, and getting some cardio and resistance training daily.
- If you want to get fit you must eat right and exercise. Similarly...
- If you want to reduce stress, you need to massage your muscles, perform antifrailty, and use breathing exercises.
- Find a group workout class in your neighborhood to attend. Make it a goal to try several of the following in the next year: cardio kickboxing, cross fit, dance, gymnastics, martial arts, Pilates, spinning, step aerobics, swimming, tumbling, yoga, and Zumba.

How I Feel Before and After

Taking this short survey before and after a workout will help you recognize how exercise can dramatically reduce stress and improve your emotional state. You can use this inventory before and after cardiovascular exercise, weight training, sports, breathing exercises, massage, or yoga. Use a scale from 1 to 10 to indicate the extent to which each word describes how you feel at each point in time. Which exercises lead to the most improvement?

	Type of Exercise	Type of Exercise	Type of Exercise	Type of Exercise	Type of Exercise
	Date / /	Date / /	Date / /	Date / /	Date / /
1. Calm	/	/	/	/	/
2. Composed	/	/	/	/	/
3. Fatigued	/	/	/	/	/
4. Enthusiastic	/	/	/	/	/
5. Relaxed	/	/	/	/	/
6. Invigorated	/	/	/	/	/
7. Cheerful	/	/	/	/	/
8. Distressed	/	/	/	/	/
9. Revived	/	/	/	/	/
10. Weary	/	/	/	/	/

	Type of Exercise	Type of Exercise	Type of Exercise	Type of Exercise	Type of Exercise
	Date / /	Date / /	Date / /	Date / /	Date / /
1. Calm	/	/	/	/	/
2. Composed	/	/	/	/	/
3. Fatigued	/	/	/	/	/
4. Enthusiastic	/	/	/	/	/
5. Relaxed	/	/	/	/	/
6. Invigorated	/	/	/	/	/
7. Cheerful	/	/	/	/	/
8. Distressed	/	/	/	/	/
9. Revived	/	/	/	/	/
10. Weary	/	/	/	/	/

Personal Commitment Contract

Committing to a behavioral contract can be an effective behavior-modification strategy. Setting up clear, precise expectations and rewards can make it easier for some people to achieve their goals. Start by filling in the first blank below with a specific goal that is realistic and attainable. It should be something measurable that you want to either perform (a consistent exercise), or achieve (body weight goal).

I agree to maintain my personal commitment to achieving or performing the following:

_____

I will do this when:_____

How frequently:_____

To what extent:_____

I also have a goal of losing _____ pounds over the next _____ weeks. I will do this responsibly at a maximum of two pounds per week.

The corresponding body fat goal is to reach _____ % body fat within this time frame.

If I can make this happen by ____/____/____, I will reward myself with:

_____.

Signed:

_____   ____/____/____.

Witnessed by:

_____

Even if you have tried to make this change in the past, make it a priority now. Feel confident that you have the ability to achieve this goal, even if it feels challenging. Prepare yourself for the inevitable setbacks, relapses, and obstacles. Gain social support from your family and friends, and feel totally confident in your ability to make this a reality.

Weekly Exercise Tracker

Start Date: _____ End Date: _____

EXERCISE		WEEK 1	WEEK 2	WEEK 3	WEEK 4
	DATE				
	REPS/SETS	/	/	/	/
	WEIGHT				
	REPS/SETS	/	/	/	/
	WEIGHT				
	REPS/SETS	/	/	/	/
	WEIGHT				
	REPS/SETS	/	/	/	/
	WEIGHT				
	REPS/SETS	/	/	/	/
	WEIGHT				
	REPS/SETS	/	/	/	/
	WEIGHT				
	REPS/SETS	/	/	/	/
	WEIGHT				
	REPS/SETS	/	/	/	/
	WEIGHT				
	REPS/SETS	/	/	/	/
	WEIGHT				
	REPS/SETS	/	/	/	/
	WEIGHT				
	REPS/SETS	/	/	/	/
	WEIGHT				
	REPS/SETS	/	/	/	/
	WEIGHT				
	REPS/SETS	/	/	/	/
	WEIGHT				
	REPS/SETS	/	/	/	/
	WEIGHT				
	REPS/SETS	/	/	/	/
	WEIGHT				
	REPS/SETS	/	/	/	/
	WEIGHT				

Weekly Exercise Tracker

Start Date: _____ End Date: _____

EXERCISE		WEEK 5	WEEK 6	WEEK 7	WEEK 8
	DATE				
	REPS/SETS	/	/	/	/
	WEIGHT				
	REPS/SETS	/	/	/	/
	WEIGHT				
	REPS/SETS	/	/	/	/
	WEIGHT				
	REPS/SETS	/	/	/	/
	WEIGHT				
	REPS/SETS	/	/	/	/
	WEIGHT				
	REPS/SETS	/	/	/	/
	WEIGHT				
	REPS/SETS	/	/	/	/
	WEIGHT				
	REPS/SETS	/	/	/	/
	WEIGHT				
	REPS/SETS	/	/	/	/
	WEIGHT				
	REPS/SETS	/	/	/	/
	WEIGHT				
	REPS/SETS	/	/	/	/
	WEIGHT				
	REPS/SETS	/	/	/	/
	WEIGHT				
	REPS/SETS	/	/	/	/
	WEIGHT				
	REPS/SETS	/	/	/	/
	WEIGHT				
	REPS/SETS	/	/	/	/
	WEIGHT				
	REPS/SETS	/	/	/	/
	WEIGHT				
	REPS/SETS	/	/	/	/
	WEIGHT				

Weekly Exercise Tracker

Start Date: _____ End Date: _____

EXERCISE		WEEK 9	WEEK 10	WEEK 11	WEEK 12
	DATE				
	REPS/SETS	/	/	/	/
	WEIGHT				
	REPS/SETS	/	/	/	/
	WEIGHT				
	REPS/SETS	/	/	/	/
	WEIGHT				
	REPS/SETS	/	/	/	/
	WEIGHT				
	REPS/SETS	/	/	/	/
	WEIGHT				
	REPS/SETS	/	/	/	/
	WEIGHT				
	REPS/SETS	/	/	/	/
	WEIGHT				
	REPS/SETS	/	/	/	/
	WEIGHT				
	REPS/SETS	/	/	/	/
	WEIGHT				
	REPS/SETS	/	/	/	/
	WEIGHT				
	REPS/SETS	/	/	/	/
	WEIGHT				
	REPS/SETS	/	/	/	/
	WEIGHT				
	REPS/SETS	/	/	/	/
	WEIGHT				
	REPS/SETS	/	/	/	/
	WEIGHT				
	REPS/SETS	/	/	/	/
	WEIGHT				
	REPS/SETS	/	/	/	/
	WEIGHT				
	REPS/SETS	/	/	/	/
	WEIGHT				

Calendar of Goals and Achievements

Month   Year

Sun	Mon	Tue	Wed	Thurs	Fri	Sat

Calendar of Goals and Achievements

_____   _____

Month   Year

Sun	Mon	Tue	Wed	Thurs	Fri	Sat

Calendar of Goals and Achievements

_____   _____

Month   Year

Sun	Mon	Tue	Wed	Thurs	Fri	Sat

Daily Fitness Tracker   Day 1

"It does not matter how slowly you go as long as you do not stop." - Confucius

Date: _____ Start Time: _____ Finish Time: _____

Cardio Description	Duration (mins)	Heart Rate Start (bpm)	Heart Rate Max (bpm)	Total Calories Burned (kcals)	Perceived Effort 1-10

Exercise Description		Set 1	Set 2	Set 3	Set 4	Set 5
	Time/Reps					
	Type/Lbs.					
	Time/Reps					
	Type/Lbs.					
	Time/Reps					
	Type/Lbs.					
	Time/Reps					
	Type/Lbs.					
	Time/Reps					
	Type/Lbs.					
	Time/Reps					
	Type/Lbs.					

Water/Fluids (oz)	Protein (grams)	Fiber (grams)	Fat (grams)	Carbs (grams)	Sugar (grams)	Sodium (grams)	Total Calories	Body Weight

Breakfast: Lunch and Snacks: Dinner:

_____   _____   _____

_____   _____   _____

_____   _____   _____

Meditation (mins)	Breathing Ex. (mins)	Sleep (hours)	Total Steps	Exercise (mins)	Flights Climbed	Standing (hours)	Stretching (mins)	Self Massage (mins)

Thoughts and Feelings:

Daily Fitness Tracker

Day 2

Did you know? Much of the pain you feel in your body from stress is actually a form of movement hunger. Tissues deprived of blood and oxygen hurt, exercise reverses this.

Date: _____ Start Time: _____ Finish Time: _____

Cardio Description	Duration (mins)	Heart Rate Start (bpm)	Heart Rate Max (bpm)	Total Calories Burned (kcals)	Perceived Effort 1-10

Exercise Description		Set 1	Set 2	Set 3	Set 4	Set 5
	Time/Reps					
	Type/Lbs.					
	Time/Reps					
	Type/Lbs.					
	Time/Reps					
	Type/Lbs.					
	Time/Reps					
	Type/Lbs.					
	Time/Reps					
	Type/Lbs.					

Water/Fluids (oz)	Protein (grams)	Fiber (grams)	Fat (grams)	Carbs (grams)	Sugar (grams)	Sodium (grams)	Total Calories	Body Weight

Breakfast:

_____

_____

_____

Lunch and Snacks:

_____

_____

_____

Dinner:

_____

_____

_____

Meditation (mins)	Breathing Ex. (mins)	Sleep (hours)	Total Steps	Exercise (mins)	Flights Climbed	Standing (hours)	Stretching (mins)	Self Massage (mins)

Thoughts and Feelings:

Daily Fitness Tracker   Day 3

"If you want something you've never had, you must be willing to do something you've never done." – Thomas Jefferson

Date: _____ Start Time: _____ Finish Time: _____

Cardio Description	Duration (mins)	Heart Rate Start (bpm)	Heart Rate Max (bpm)	Total Calories Burned (kcals)	Perceived Effort 1-10

Exercise Description		Set 1	Set 2	Set 3	Set 4	Set 5
	Time/Reps					
	Type/Lbs.					
	Time/Reps					
	Type/Lbs.					
	Time/Reps					
	Type/Lbs.					
	Time/Reps					
	Type/Lbs.					
	Time/Reps					
	Type/Lbs.					
	Time/Reps					
	Type/Lbs.					

Water/Fluids (oz)	Protein (grams)	Fiber (grams)	Fat (grams)	Carbs (grams)	Sugar (grams)	Sodium (grams)	Total Calories	Body Weight

Breakfast: Lunch and Snacks: Dinner:

_____   _____   _____

_____   _____   _____

_____   _____   _____

Meditation (mins)	Breathing Ex. (mins)	Sleep (hours)	Total Steps	Exercise (mins)	Flights Climbed	Standing (hours)	Stretching (mins)	Self Massage (mins)

Thoughts and Feelings:

Daily Fitness Tracker   Day 4

"Food and exercise work together to produce health." – Hippocrates

Date: _____ Start Time: _____ Finish Time: _____

Cardio Description	Duration (mins)	Heart Rate Start (bpm)	Heart Rate Max (bpm)	Total Calories Burned (kcals)	Perceived Effort 1-10

Exercise Description		Set 1	Set 2	Set 3	Set 4	Set 5
	Time/Reps					
	Type/Lbs.					
	Time/Reps					
	Type/Lbs.					
	Time/Reps					
	Type/Lbs.					
	Time/Reps					
	Type/Lbs.					
	Time/Reps					
	Type/Lbs.					
	Time/Reps					
	Type/Lbs.					

Water/Fluids (oz)	Protein (grams)	Fiber (grams)	Fat (grams)	Carbs (grams)	Sugar (grams)	Sodium (grams)	Total Calories	Body Weight

Breakfast: Lunch and Snacks: Dinner:

_____   _____   _____

_____   _____   _____

_____   _____   _____

Meditation (mins)	Breathing Ex. (mins)	Sleep (hours)	Total Steps	Exercise (mins)	Flights Climbed	Standing (hours)	Stretching (mins)	Self Massage (mins)

Thoughts and Feelings:

Daily Fitness Tracker   Day 5

"Once you are doing exercise regularly, the hardest thing is to stop it." – Erin Gray

Date: _____ Start Time: _____ Finish Time: _____

Cardio Description	Duration (mins)	Heart Rate Start (bpm)	Heart Rate Max (bpm)	Total Calories Burned (kcals)	Perceived Effort 1-10

Exercise Description		Set 1	Set 2	Set 3	Set 4	Set 5
	Time/Reps					
	Type/Lbs.					
	Time/Reps					
	Type/Lbs.					
	Time/Reps					
	Type/Lbs.					
	Time/Reps					
	Type/Lbs.					
	Time/Reps					
	Type/Lbs.					
	Time/Reps					
	Type/Lbs.					

Water/Fluids (oz)	Protein (grams)	Fiber (grams)	Fat (grams)	Carbs (grams)	Sugar (grams)	Sodium (grams)	Total Calories	Body Weight

Breakfast: Lunch and Snacks: Dinner:

_____   _____   _____

_____   _____   _____

_____   _____   _____

Meditation (mins)	Breathing Ex. (mins)	Sleep (hours)	Total Steps	Exercise (mins)	Flights Climbed	Standing (hours)	Stretching (mins)	Self Massage (mins)

Thoughts and Feelings:

Daily Fitness Tracker   Day 6

"If it doesn't challenge you, it doesn't change you." – Kenneth H. Cooper

Date: _____ Start Time: _____ Finish Time: _____

Cardio Description	Duration (mins)	Heart Rate Start (bpm)	Heart Rate Max (bpm)	Total Calories Burned (kcals)	Perceived Effort 1-10

Exercise Description		Set 1	Set 2	Set 3	Set 4	Set 5
	Time/Reps					
	Type/Lbs.					
	Time/Reps					
	Type/Lbs.					
	Time/Reps					
	Type/Lbs.					
	Time/Reps					
	Type/Lbs.					
	Time/Reps					
	Type/Lbs.					
	Time/Reps					
	Type/Lbs.					

Water/Fluids (oz)	Protein (grams)	Fiber (grams)	Fat (grams)	Carbs (grams)	Sugar (grams)	Sodium (grams)	Total Calories	Body Weight

Breakfast: Lunch and Snacks: Dinner:

_____   _____   _____

_____   _____   _____

_____   _____   _____

Meditation (mins)	Breathing Ex. (mins)	Sleep (hours)	Total Steps	Exercise (mins)	Flights Climbed	Standing (hours)	Stretching (mins)	Self Massage (mins)

Thoughts and Feelings:

Daily Fitness Tracker   Day 7

Did you know? A one hour workout is only 4% of your day.

Date: _____ Start Time: _____ Finish Time: _____

Cardio Description	Duration (mins)	Heart Rate Start (bpm)	Heart Rate Max (bpm)	Total Calories Burned (kcals)	Perceived Effort 1-10

Exercise Description		Set 1	Set 2	Set 3	Set 4	Set 5
	Time/Reps					
	Type/Lbs.					
	Time/Reps					
	Type/Lbs.					
	Time/Reps					
	Type/Lbs.					
	Time/Reps					
	Type/Lbs.					
	Time/Reps					
	Type/Lbs.					
	Time/Reps					
	Type/Lbs.					

Water/Fluids (oz)	Protein (grams)	Fiber (grams)	Fat (grams)	Carbs (grams)	Sugar (grams)	Sodium (grams)	Total Calories	Body Weight

Breakfast: Lunch and Snacks: Dinner:

_____   _____   _____

_____   _____   _____

_____   _____   _____

Meditation (mins)	Breathing Ex. (mins)	Sleep (hours)	Total Steps	Exercise (mins)	Flights Climbed	Standing (hours)	Stretching (mins)	Self Massage (mins)

Thoughts and Feelings:

Daily Fitness Tracker

Day 8

"Exercise is about as close to a magic potion as you can get." – Tich Nhat Hanh

Date: _____ Start Time: _____ Finish Time: _____

Cardio Description	Duration (mins)	Heart Rate Start (bpm)	Heart Rate Max (bpm)	Total Calories Burned (kcals)	Perceived Effort 1-10

Exercise Description		Set 1	Set 2	Set 3	Set 4	Set 5
	Time/Reps					
	Type/Lbs.					
	Time/Reps					
	Type/Lbs.					
	Time/Reps					
	Type/Lbs.					
	Time/Reps					
	Type/Lbs.					
	Time/Reps					
	Type/Lbs.					
	Time/Reps					
	Type/Lbs.					

Water/Fluids (oz)	Protein (grams)	Fiber (grams)	Fat (grams)	Carbs (grams)	Sugar (grams)	Sodium (grams)	Total Calories	Body Weight

Breakfast: Lunch and Snacks: Dinner:

_____   _____   _____

_____   _____   _____

_____   _____   _____

Meditation (mins)	Breathing Ex. (mins)	Sleep (hours)	Total Steps	Exercise (mins)	Flights Climbed	Standing (hours)	Stretching (mins)	Self Massage (mins)

Thoughts and Feelings:

Daily Fitness Tracker   Day 9

"The best time to plant a tree is 20 years ago. The second best time is now." –Proverb

Date: _____ Start Time: _____ Finish Time: _____

Cardio Description	Duration (mins)	Heart Rate Start (bpm)	Heart Rate Max (bpm)	Total Calories Burned (kcals)	Perceived Effort 1-10

Exercise Description		Set 1	Set 2	Set 3	Set 4	Set 5
	Time/Reps					
	Type/Lbs.					
	Time/Reps					
	Type/Lbs.					
	Time/Reps					
	Type/Lbs.					
	Time/Reps					
	Type/Lbs.					
	Time/Reps					
	Type/Lbs.					
	Time/Reps					
	Type/Lbs.					

Water/Fluids (oz)	Protein (grams)	Fiber (grams)	Fat (grams)	Carbs (grams)	Sugar (grams)	Sodium (grams)	Total Calories	Body Weight

Breakfast: Lunch and Snacks: Dinner:

_____   _____   _____

_____   _____   _____

_____   _____   _____

Meditation (mins)	Breathing Ex. (mins)	Sleep (hours)	Total Steps	Exercise (mins)	Flights Climbed	Standing (hours)	Stretching (mins)	Self Massage (mins)

Thoughts and Feelings:

Daily Fitness Tracker   # Day 10

"If you don't make time for exercise, you'll probably have to make time for illness." – R. Sharma

Date: _____ Start Time: _____ Finish Time: _____

Cardio Description	Duration (mins)	Heart Rate Start (bpm)	Heart Rate Max (bpm)	Total Calories Burned (kcals)	Perceived Effort 1-10

Exercise Description		Set 1	Set 2	Set 3	Set 4	Set 5
	Time/Reps					
	Type/Lbs.					
	Time/Reps					
	Type/Lbs.					
	Time/Reps					
	Type/Lbs.					
	Time/Reps					
	Type/Lbs.					
	Time/Reps					
	Type/Lbs.					
	Time/Reps					
	Type/Lbs.					

Water/Fluids (oz)	Protein (grams)	Fiber (grams)	Fat (grams)	Carbs (grams)	Sugar (grams)	Sodium (grams)	Total Calories	Body Weight

Breakfast: Lunch and Snacks: Dinner:

_____   _____   _____

_____   _____   _____

_____   _____   _____

Meditation (mins)	Breathing Ex. (mins)	Sleep (hours)	Total Steps	Exercise (mins)	Flights Climbed	Standing (hours)	Stretching (mins)	Self Massage (mins)

Thoughts and Feelings:

Daily Fitness Tracker   # Day 11

"Walking is the best possible exercise. Habituate yourself to walk very far." – Thomas Jefferson

Date: _____ Start Time: _____ Finish Time: _____

Cardio Description	Duration (mins)	Heart Rate Start (bpm)	Heart Rate Max (bpm)	Total Calories Burned (kcals)	Perceived Effort 1-10

Exercise Description		Set 1	Set 2	Set 3	Set 4	Set 5
	Time/Reps					
	Type/Lbs.					
	Time/Reps					
	Type/Lbs.					
	Time/Reps					
	Type/Lbs.					
	Time/Reps					
	Type/Lbs.					
	Time/Reps					
	Type/Lbs.					
	Time/Reps					
	Type/Lbs.					

Water/Fluids (oz)	Protein (grams)	Fiber (grams)	Fat (grams)	Carbs (grams)	Sugar (grams)	Sodium (grams)	Total Calories	Body Weight

Breakfast: Lunch and Snacks: Dinner:

_____   _____   _____

_____   _____   _____

_____   _____   _____

Meditation (mins)	Breathing Ex. (mins)	Sleep (hours)	Total Steps	Exercise (mins)	Flights Climbed	Standing (hours)	Stretching (mins)	Self Massage (mins)

Thoughts and Feelings:

Daily Fitness Tracker

Day 12

"Exercise is psychological therapy." – Anonymous

Date: _____ Start Time: _____ Finish Time: _____

Cardio Description	Duration (mins)	Heart Rate Start (bpm)	Heart Rate Max (bpm)	Total Calories Burned (kcals)	Perceived Effort 1-10

Exercise Description		Set 1	Set 2	Set 3	Set 4	Set 5
	Time/Reps					
	Type/Lbs.					
	Time/Reps					
	Type/Lbs.					
	Time/Reps					
	Type/Lbs.					
	Time/Reps					
	Type/Lbs.					
	Time/Reps					
	Type/Lbs.					
	Time/Reps					
	Type/Lbs.					

Water/Fluids (oz)	Protein (grams)	Fiber (grams)	Fat (grams)	Carbs (grams)	Sugar (grams)	Sodium (grams)	Total Calories	Body Weight

Breakfast:

_____

_____

_____

Lunch and Snacks:

_____

_____

_____

Dinner:

_____

_____

_____

Meditation (mins)	Breathing Ex. (mins)	Sleep (hours)	Total Steps	Exercise (mins)	Flights Climbed	Standing (hours)	Stretching (mins)	Self Massage (mins)

Thoughts and Feelings:

Daily Fitness Tracker   **Day 13**

"The most difficult thing is the decision to act, the rest is merely tenacity." – Amelia Earhart

Date: _____ Start Time: _____ Finish Time: _____

Cardio Description	Duration (mins)	Heart Rate Start (bpm)	Heart Rate Max (bpm)	Total Calories Burned (kcals)	Perceived Effort 1-10

Exercise Description		Set 1	Set 2	Set 3	Set 4	Set 5
	Time/Reps					
	Type/Lbs.					
	Time/Reps					
	Type/Lbs.					
	Time/Reps					
	Type/Lbs.					
	Time/Reps					
	Type/Lbs.					
	Time/Reps					
	Type/Lbs.					
	Time/Reps					
	Type/Lbs.					

Water/Fluids (oz)	Protein (grams)	Fiber (grams)	Fat (grams)	Carbs (grams)	Sugar (grams)	Sodium (grams)	Total Calories	Body Weight

Breakfast: Lunch and Snacks: Dinner:

_____   _____   _____

_____   _____   _____

_____   _____   _____

Meditation (mins)	Breathing Ex. (mins)	Sleep (hours)	Total Steps	Exercise (mins)	Flights Climbed	Standing (hours)	Stretching (mins)	Self Massage (mins)

Thoughts and Feelings:

Daily Fitness Tracker   **Day 14**

"Step into the new story you are willing to create." – Oprah Winfrey

Date: _____ Start Time: _____ Finish Time: _____

Cardio Description	Duration (mins)	Heart Rate Start (bpm)	Heart Rate Max (bpm)	Total Calories Burned (kcals)	Perceived Effort 1-10

Exercise Description		Set 1	Set 2	Set 3	Set 4	Set 5
	Time/Reps					
	Type/Lbs.					
	Time/Reps					
	Type/Lbs.					
	Time/Reps					
	Type/Lbs.					
	Time/Reps					
	Type/Lbs.					
	Time/Reps					
	Type/Lbs.					
	Time/Reps					
	Type/Lbs.					

Water/Fluids (oz)	Protein (grams)	Fiber (grams)	Fat (grams)	Carbs (grams)	Sugar (grams)	Sodium (grams)	Total Calories	Body Weight

Breakfast: Lunch and Snacks: Dinner:

_____   _____   _____

_____   _____   _____

_____   _____   _____

Meditation (mins)	Breathing Ex. (mins)	Sleep (hours)	Total Steps	Exercise (mins)	Flights Climbed	Standing (hours)	Stretching (mins)	Self Massage (mins)

Thoughts and Feelings:

Daily Fitness Tracker   Day 15

"It is exercise alone that supports the spirits, and keeps the mind in vigor." – Marcus Cicero

Date: _____ Start Time: _____ Finish Time: _____

Cardio Description	Duration (mins)	Heart Rate Start (bpm)	Heart Rate Max (bpm)	Total Calories Burned (kcals)	Perceived Effort 1-10

Exercise Description		Set 1	Set 2	Set 3	Set 4	Set 5
	Time/Reps					
	Type/Lbs.					
	Time/Reps					
	Type/Lbs.					
	Time/Reps					
	Type/Lbs.					
	Time/Reps					
	Type/Lbs.					
	Time/Reps					
	Type/Lbs.					
	Time/Reps					
	Type/Lbs.					

Water/Fluids (oz)	Protein (grams)	Fiber (grams)	Fat (grams)	Carbs (grams)	Sugar (grams)	Sodium (grams)	Total Calories	Body Weight

Breakfast: Lunch and Snacks: Dinner:

_____   _____   _____

_____   _____   _____

_____   _____   _____

Meditation (mins)	Breathing Ex. (mins)	Sleep (hours)	Total Steps	Exercise (mins)	Flights Climbed	Standing (hours)	Stretching (mins)	Self Massage (mins)

Thoughts and Feelings:

Daily Fitness Tracker   **Day 16**

"Lack of activity destroys the good condition of every human being." – Plato

Date: _____ Start Time: _____ Finish Time: _____

Cardio Description	Duration (mins)	Heart Rate Start (bpm)	Heart Rate Max (bpm)	Total Calories Burned (kcals)	Perceived Effort 1-10

Exercise Description		Set 1	Set 2	Set 3	Set 4	Set 5
	Time/Reps					
	Type/Lbs.					
	Time/Reps					
	Type/Lbs.					
	Time/Reps					
	Type/Lbs.					
	Time/Reps					
	Type/Lbs.					
	Time/Reps					
	Type/Lbs.					
	Time/Reps					
	Type/Lbs.					

Water/Fluids (oz)	Protein (grams)	Fiber (grams)	Fat (grams)	Carbs (grams)	Sugar (grams)	Sodium (grams)	Total Calories	Body Weight

Breakfast: Lunch and Snacks: Dinner:

_____   _____   _____

_____   _____   _____

_____   _____   _____

Meditation (mins)	Breathing Ex. (mins)	Sleep (hours)	Total Steps	Exercise (mins)	Flights Climbed	Standing (hours)	Stretching (mins)	Self Massage (mins)

Thoughts and Feelings:

Daily Fitness Tracker   # Day 17

"Great effort is required to arrest decay and restore vigor." – Horace

Date: _____ Start Time: _____ Finish Time: _____

Cardio Description	Duration (mins)	Heart Rate Start (bpm)	Heart Rate Max (bpm)	Total Calories Burned (kcals)	Perceived Effort 1-10

Exercise Description		Set 1	Set 2	Set 3	Set 4	Set 5
	Time/Reps					
	Type/Lbs.					
	Time/Reps					
	Type/Lbs.					
	Time/Reps					
	Type/Lbs.					
	Time/Reps					
	Type/Lbs.					
	Time/Reps					
	Type/Lbs.					
	Time/Reps					
	Type/Lbs.					

Water/Fluids (oz)	Protein (grams)	Fiber (grams)	Fat (grams)	Carbs (grams)	Sugar (grams)	Sodium (grams)	Total Calories	Body Weight

Breakfast: Lunch and Snacks: Dinner:

_____   _____   _____

_____   _____   _____

_____   _____   _____

Meditation (mins)	Breathing Ex. (mins)	Sleep (hours)	Total Steps	Exercise (mins)	Flights Climbed	Standing (hours)	Stretching (mins)	Self Massage (mins)

Thoughts and Feelings:

Daily Fitness Tracker   Day 18

"Nothing lifts me out of a bad mood better than a hard work out on my treadmill." – Cher

Date: _____ Start Time: _____ Finish Time: _____

Cardio Description	Duration (mins)	Heart Rate Start (bpm)	Heart Rate Max (bpm)	Total Calories Burned (kcals)	Perceived Effort 1-10

Exercise Description		Set 1	Set 2	Set 3	Set 4	Set 5
	Time/Reps					
	Type/Lbs.					
	Time/Reps					
	Type/Lbs.					
	Time/Reps					
	Type/Lbs.					
	Time/Reps					
	Type/Lbs.					
	Time/Reps					
	Type/Lbs.					
	Time/Reps					
	Type/Lbs.					

Water/Fluids (oz)	Protein (grams)	Fiber (grams)	Fat (grams)	Carbs (grams)	Sugar (grams)	Sodium (grams)	Total Calories	Body Weight

Breakfast: Lunch and Snacks: Dinner:

_____   _____   _____

_____   _____   _____

_____   _____   _____

Meditation (mins)	Breathing Ex. (mins)	Sleep (hours)	Total Steps	Exercise (mins)	Flights Climbed	Standing (hours)	Stretching (mins)	Self Massage (mins)

Thoughts and Feelings:

Daily Fitness Tracker   **Day 19**

"An early-morning walk is a blessing for the whole day." – Adam Smith

Date: _____ Start Time: _____ Finish Time: _____

Cardio Description	Duration (mins)	Heart Rate Start (bpm)	Heart Rate Max (bpm)	Total Calories Burned (kcals)	Perceived Effort 1-10

Exercise Description		Set 1	Set 2	Set 3	Set 4	Set 5
	Time/Reps					
	Type/Lbs.					
	Time/Reps					
	Type/Lbs.					
	Time/Reps					
	Type/Lbs.					
	Time/Reps					
	Type/Lbs.					
	Time/Reps					
	Type/Lbs.					
	Time/Reps					
	Type/Lbs.					

Water/Fluids (oz)	Protein (grams)	Fiber (grams)	Fat (grams)	Carbs (grams)	Sugar (grams)	Sodium (grams)	Total Calories	Body Weight

Breakfast: Lunch and Snacks: Dinner:

_____   _____   _____

_____   _____   _____

_____   _____   _____

Meditation (mins)	Breathing Ex. (mins)	Sleep (hours)	Total Steps	Exercise (mins)	Flights Climbed	Standing (hours)	Stretching (mins)	Self Massage (mins)

Thoughts and Feelings:

Daily Fitness Tracker   **Day 20**

"Physical fitness… is the basis of dynamic and creative intellectual activity." – John F. Kennedy

Date: _____ Start Time: _____ Finish Time: _____

Cardio Description	Duration (mins)	Heart Rate Start (bpm)	Heart Rate Max (bpm)	Total Calories Burned (kcals)	Perceived Effort 1-10

Exercise Description		Set 1	Set 2	Set 3	Set 4	Set 5
	Time/Reps					
	Type/Lbs.					
	Time/Reps					
	Type/Lbs.					
	Time/Reps					
	Type/Lbs.					
	Time/Reps					
	Type/Lbs.					
	Time/Reps					
	Type/Lbs.					
	Time/Reps					
	Type/Lbs.					

Water/Fluids (oz)	Protein (grams)	Fiber (grams)	Fat (grams)	Carbs (grams)	Sugar (grams)	Sodium (grams)	Total Calories	Body Weight

Breakfast: Lunch and Snacks: Dinner:

_____   _____   _____

_____   _____   _____

_____   _____   _____

Meditation (mins)	Breathing Ex. (mins)	Sleep (hours)	Total Steps	Exercise (mins)	Flights Climbed	Standing (hours)	Stretching (mins)	Self Massage (mins)

Thoughts and Feelings:

Daily Fitness Tracker   **Day 21**

"We do not stop exercising because we grow old - we grow old because we stop exercising."

Date: _____ Start Time: _____ Finish Time: _____

Cardio Description	Duration (mins)	Heart Rate Start (bpm)	Heart Rate Max (bpm)	Total Calories Burned (kcals)	Perceived Effort 1-10

Exercise Description		Set 1	Set 2	Set 3	Set 4	Set 5
	Time/Reps					
	Type/Lbs.					
	Time/Reps					
	Type/Lbs.					
	Time/Reps					
	Type/Lbs.					
	Time/Reps					
	Type/Lbs.					
	Time/Reps					
	Type/Lbs.					
	Time/Reps					
	Type/Lbs.					

Water/Fluids (oz)	Protein (grams)	Fiber (grams)	Fat (grams)	Carbs (grams)	Sugar (grams)	Sodium (grams)	Total Calories	Body Weight

Breakfast: Lunch and Snacks: Dinner:

_____   _____   _____

_____   _____   _____

_____   _____   _____

Meditation (mins)	Breathing Ex. (mins)	Sleep (hours)	Total Steps	Exercise (mins)	Flights Climbed	Standing (hours)	Stretching (mins)	Self Massage (mins)

Thoughts and Feelings:

Daily Fitness Tracker   **Day 22**

"Movement is a medicine for creating change in a person's physical, emotional, and mental states." – Carol Welch

Date: _____ Start Time: _____ Finish Time: _____

Cardio Description	Duration (mins)	Heart Rate Start (bpm)	Heart Rate Max (bpm)	Total Calories Burned (kcals)	Perceived Effort 1-10

Exercise Description		Set 1	Set 2	Set 3	Set 4	Set 5
	Time/Reps					
	Type/Lbs.					
	Time/Reps					
	Type/Lbs.					
	Time/Reps					
	Type/Lbs.					
	Time/Reps					
	Type/Lbs.					
	Time/Reps					
	Type/Lbs.					
	Time/Reps					
	Type/Lbs.					

Water/Fluids (oz)	Protein (grams)	Fiber (grams)	Fat (grams)	Carbs (grams)	Sugar (grams)	Sodium (grams)	Total Calories	Body Weight

Breakfast: Lunch and Snacks: Dinner:

_____   _____   _____

_____   _____   _____

_____   _____   _____

Meditation (mins)	Breathing Ex. (mins)	Sleep (hours)	Total Steps	Exercise (mins)	Flights Climbed	Standing (hours)	Stretching (mins)	Self Massage (mins)

Thoughts and Feelings:

Daily Fitness Tracker   Day 23

"It is a shame for a man to grow old without seeing the beauty and strength of which his body is capable." – Socrates

Date: _____ Start Time: _____ Finish Time: _____

Cardio Description	Duration (mins)	Heart Rate Start (bpm)	Heart Rate Max (bpm)	Total Calories Burned (kcals)	Perceived Effort 1-10

Exercise Description		Set 1	Set 2	Set 3	Set 4	Set 5
	Time/Reps					
	Type/Lbs.					
	Time/Reps					
	Type/Lbs.					
	Time/Reps					
	Type/Lbs.					
	Time/Reps					
	Type/Lbs.					
	Time/Reps					
	Type/Lbs.					
	Time/Reps					
	Type/Lbs.					

Water/Fluids (oz)	Protein (grams)	Fiber (grams)	Fat (grams)	Carbs (grams)	Sugar (grams)	Sodium (grams)	Total Calories	Body Weight

Breakfast: Lunch and Snacks: Dinner:

_____   _____   _____

_____   _____   _____

_____   _____   _____

Meditation (mins)	Breathing Ex. (mins)	Sleep (hours)	Total Steps	Exercise (mins)	Flights Climbed	Standing (hours)	Stretching (mins)	Self Massage (mins)

Thoughts and Feelings:

Daily Fitness Tracker

Day 24

"Other exercises develop single powers and muscles, but dancing embellishes, exercises, and equalizes all the muscles at once. – Jean Paul

Date: _____ Start Time: _____ Finish Time: _____

Cardio Description	Duration (mins)	Heart Rate Start (bpm)	Heart Rate Max (bpm)	Total Calories Burned (kcals)	Perceived Effort 1-10

Exercise Description		Set 1	Set 2	Set 3	Set 4	Set 5
	Time/Reps					
	Type/Lbs.					
	Time/Reps					
	Type/Lbs.					
	Time/Reps					
	Type/Lbs.					
	Time/Reps					
	Type/Lbs.					
	Time/Reps					
	Type/Lbs.					
	Time/Reps					
	Type/Lbs.					

Water/Fluids (oz)	Protein (grams)	Fiber (grams)	Fat (grams)	Carbs (grams)	Sugar (grams)	Sodium (grams)	Total Calories	Body Weight

Breakfast:

_____
_____
_____

Lunch and Snacks:

_____
_____
_____

Dinner:

_____
_____
_____

Meditation (mins)	Breathing Ex. (mins)	Sleep (hours)	Total Steps	Exercise (mins)	Flights Climbed	Standing (hours)	Stretching (mins)	Self Massage (mins)

Thoughts and Feelings:

Daily Fitness Tracker   **Day 25**

"Training gives us an outlet for suppressed energies created by stress and thus tones the spirit just as exercise conditions the body." – Arnold Schwarzenegger

Date: _____ Start Time: _____ Finish Time: _____

Cardio Description	Duration (mins)	Heart Rate Start (bpm)	Heart Rate Max (bpm)	Total Calories Burned (kcals)	Perceived Effort 1-10

Exercise Description		Set 1	Set 2	Set 3	Set 4	Set 5
	Time/Reps					
	Type/Lbs.					
	Time/Reps					
	Type/Lbs.					
	Time/Reps					
	Type/Lbs.					
	Time/Reps					
	Type/Lbs.					
	Time/Reps					
	Type/Lbs.					
	Time/Reps					
	Type/Lbs.					

Water/Fluids (oz)	Protein (grams)	Fiber (grams)	Fat (grams)	Carbs (grams)	Sugar (grams)	Sodium (grams)	Total Calories	Body Weight

Breakfast: Lunch and Snacks: Dinner:

_____   _____   _____

_____   _____   _____

_____   _____   _____

Meditation (mins)	Breathing Ex. (mins)	Sleep (hours)	Total Steps	Exercise (mins)	Flights Climbed	Standing (hours)	Stretching (mins)	Self Massage (mins)

Thoughts and Feelings:

Daily Fitness Tracker   **Day 26**

"Exercise to stimulate, not to annihilate. The world wasn't formed in a day, and neither were we. Set small goals and build upon them." – Lee Haney

Date: _____ Start Time: _____ Finish Time: _____

Cardio Description	Duration (mins)	Heart Rate Start (bpm)	Heart Rate Max (bpm)	Total Calories Burned (kcals)	Perceived Effort 1-10

Exercise Description		Set 1	Set 2	Set 3	Set 4	Set 5
	Time/Reps					
	Type/Lbs.					
	Time/Reps					
	Type/Lbs.					
	Time/Reps					
	Type/Lbs.					
	Time/Reps					
	Type/Lbs.					
	Time/Reps					
	Type/Lbs.					
	Time/Reps					
	Type/Lbs.					

Water/Fluids (oz)	Protein (grams)	Fiber (grams)	Fat (grams)	Carbs (grams)	Sugar (grams)	Sodium (grams)	Total Calories	Body Weight

Breakfast: Lunch and Snacks: Dinner:

_____   _____   _____

_____   _____   _____

_____   _____   _____

Meditation (mins)	Breathing Ex. (mins)	Sleep (hours)	Total Steps	Exercise (mins)	Flights Climbed	Standing (hours)	Stretching (mins)	Self Massage (mins)

Thoughts and Feelings:

Daily Fitness Tracker   **Day 27**

"True enjoyment comes from activity of the mind and exercise of the body; the two are ever united." – Wilhelm Von Helmboldt

Date: _____ Start Time: _____ Finish Time: _____

Cardio Description	Duration (mins)	Heart Rate Start (bpm)	Heart Rate Max (bpm)	Total Calories Burned (kcals)	Perceived Effort 1-10

Exercise Description		Set 1	Set 2	Set 3	Set 4	Set 5
	Time/Reps					
	Type/Lbs.					
	Time/Reps					
	Type/Lbs.					
	Time/Reps					
	Type/Lbs.					
	Time/Reps					
	Type/Lbs.					
	Time/Reps					
	Type/Lbs.					
	Time/Reps					
	Type/Lbs.					

Water/Fluids (oz)	Protein (grams)	Fiber (grams)	Fat (grams)	Carbs (grams)	Sugar (grams)	Sodium (grams)	Total Calories	Body Weight

Breakfast: Lunch and Snacks: Dinner:

_____   _____   _____

_____   _____   _____

_____   _____   _____

Meditation (mins)	Breathing Ex. (mins)	Sleep (hours)	Total Steps	Exercise (mins)	Flights Climbed	Standing (hours)	Stretching (mins)	Self Massage (mins)

Thoughts and Feelings:

Daily Fitness Tracker   **Day 28**

"Obstacles are what you see when you take your eye off the goal." – Chris Burke

Date: _____ Start Time: _____ Finish Time: _____

Cardio Description	Duration (mins)	Heart Rate Start (bpm)	Heart Rate Max (bpm)	Total Calories Burned (kcals)	Perceived Effort 1-10

Exercise Description		Set 1	Set 2	Set 3	Set 4	Set 5
	Time/Reps					
	Type/Lbs.					
	Time/Reps					
	Type/Lbs.					
	Time/Reps					
	Type/Lbs.					
	Time/Reps					
	Type/Lbs.					
	Time/Reps					
	Type/Lbs.					

Water/Fluids (oz)	Protein (grams)	Fiber (grams)	Fat (grams)	Carbs (grams)	Sugar (grams)	Sodium (grams)	Total Calories	Body Weight

Breakfast: Lunch and Snacks: Dinner:

_____   _____   _____

_____   _____   _____

_____   _____   _____

Meditation (mins)	Breathing Ex. (mins)	Sleep (hours)	Total Steps	Exercise (mins)	Flights Climbed	Standing (hours)	Stretching (mins)	Self Massage (mins)

Thoughts and Feelings:

Daily Fitness Tracker   Day 29

"A year from now you may wish you had started today." – Karen Lamb

Date: _____ Start Time: _____ Finish Time: _____

Cardio Description	Duration (mins)	Heart Rate Start (bpm)	Heart Rate Max (bpm)	Total Calories Burned (kcals)	Perceived Effort 1-10

Exercise Description		Set 1	Set 2	Set 3	Set 4	Set 5
	Time/Reps					
	Type/Lbs.					
	Time/Reps					
	Type/Lbs.					
	Time/Reps					
	Type/Lbs.					
	Time/Reps					
	Type/Lbs.					
	Time/Reps					
	Type/Lbs.					
	Time/Reps					
	Type/Lbs.					

Water/Fluids (oz)	Protein (grams)	Fiber (grams)	Fat (grams)	Carbs (grams)	Sugar (grams)	Sodium (grams)	Total Calories	Body Weight

Breakfast: Lunch and Snacks: Dinner:

_____   _____   _____

_____   _____   _____

_____   _____   _____

Meditation (mins)	Breathing Ex. (mins)	Sleep (hours)	Total Steps	Exercise (mins)	Flights Climbed	Standing (hours)	Stretching (mins)	Self Massage (mins)

Thoughts and Feelings:

Daily Fitness Tracker   **Day 30**

"Obstacles can't stop you. Problems can't stop you. Most of all, other people can't stop you. Only you can stop you." – Amelia Earhart

Date: _____ Start Time: _____ Finish Time: _____

Cardio Description	Duration (mins)	Heart Rate Start (bpm)	Heart Rate Max (bpm)	Total Calories Burned (kcals)	Perceived Effort 1-10

Exercise Description		Set 1	Set 2	Set 3	Set 4	Set 5
	Time/Reps					
	Type/Lbs.					
	Time/Reps					
	Type/Lbs.					
	Time/Reps					
	Type/Lbs.					
	Time/Reps					
	Type/Lbs.					
	Time/Reps					
	Type/Lbs.					
	Time/Reps					
	Type/Lbs.					

Water/Fluids (oz)	Protein (grams)	Fiber (grams)	Fat (grams)	Carbs (grams)	Sugar (grams)	Sodium (grams)	Total Calories	Body Weight

Breakfast: Lunch and Snacks: Dinner:

_____   _____   _____

_____   _____   _____

_____   _____   _____

Meditation (mins)	Breathing Ex. (mins)	Sleep (hours)	Total Steps	Exercise (mins)	Flights Climbed	Standing (hours)	Stretching (mins)	Self Massage (mins)

Thoughts and Feelings:

Daily Fitness Tracker   **Day 31**

"Winners are losers who got up and gave it one more try." – Dennis DeYoung

Date: _____ Start Time: _____ Finish Time: _____

Cardio Description	Duration (mins)	Heart Rate Start (bpm)	Heart Rate Max (bpm)	Total Calories Burned (kcals)	Perceived Effort 1-10

Exercise Description		Set 1	Set 2	Set 3	Set 4	Set 5
	Time/Reps					
	Type/Lbs.					
	Time/Reps					
	Type/Lbs.					
	Time/Reps					
	Type/Lbs.					
	Time/Reps					
	Type/Lbs.					
	Time/Reps					
	Type/Lbs.					
	Time/Reps					
	Type/Lbs.					

Water/Fluids (oz)	Protein (grams)	Fiber (grams)	Fat (grams)	Carbs (grams)	Sugar (grams)	Sodium (grams)	Total Calories	Body Weight

Breakfast: Lunch and Snacks: Dinner:

_____   _____   _____

_____   _____   _____

_____   _____   _____

Meditation (mins)	Breathing Ex. (mins)	Sleep (hours)	Total Steps	Exercise (mins)	Flights Climbed	Standing (hours)	Stretching (mins)	Self Massage (mins)

Thoughts and Feelings:

Daily Fitness Tracker

Day 32

Did you know? Exercise increases energy levels, and mental clarity by increasing levels of the brain chemical serotonin.

Date: _____ Start Time: _____ Finish Time: _____

Cardio Description	Duration (mins)	Heart Rate Start (bpm)	Heart Rate Max (bpm)	Total Calories Burned (kcals)	Perceived Effort 1-10

Exercise Description		Set 1	Set 2	Set 3	Set 4	Set 5
	Time/Reps					
	Type/Lbs.					
	Time/Reps					
	Type/Lbs.					
	Time/Reps					
	Type/Lbs.					
	Time/Reps					
	Type/Lbs.					
	Time/Reps					
	Type/Lbs.					
	Time/Reps					
	Type/Lbs.					

Water/Fluids (oz)	Protein (grams)	Fiber (grams)	Fat (grams)	Carbs (grams)	Sugar (grams)	Sodium (grams)	Total Calories	Body Weight

Breakfast: Lunch and Snacks: Dinner:

_____   _____   _____

_____   _____   _____

_____   _____   _____

Meditation (mins)	Breathing Ex. (mins)	Sleep (hours)	Total Steps	Exercise (mins)	Flights Climbed	Standing (hours)	Stretching (mins)	Self Massage (mins)

Thoughts and Feelings:

Daily Fitness Tracker   **Day 33**

Did you know? People that exercise and stay active are more productive at work.

Date: _____ Start Time: _____ Finish Time: _____

Cardio Description	Duration (mins)	Heart Rate Start (bpm)	Heart Rate Max (bpm)	Total Calories Burned (kcals)	Perceived Effort 1-10

Exercise Description		Set 1	Set 2	Set 3	Set 4	Set 5
	Time/Reps					
	Type/Lbs.					
	Time/Reps					
	Type/Lbs.					
	Time/Reps					
	Type/Lbs.					
	Time/Reps					
	Type/Lbs.					
	Time/Reps					
	Type/Lbs.					
	Time/Reps					
	Type/Lbs.					

Water/Fluids (oz)	Protein (grams)	Fiber (grams)	Fat (grams)	Carbs (grams)	Sugar (grams)	Sodium (grams)	Total Calories	Body Weight

Breakfast: Lunch and Snacks: Dinner:

_____   _____   _____

_____   _____   _____

_____   _____   _____

Meditation (mins)	Breathing Ex. (mins)	Sleep (hours)	Total Steps	Exercise (mins)	Flights Climbed	Standing (hours)	Stretching (mins)	Self Massage (mins)

Thoughts and Feelings:

Daily Fitness Tracker   **Day 34**

Did you know? Exercise produces a relaxation response that melts away stress.

Date: _____ Start Time: _____ Finish Time: _____

Cardio Description	Duration (mins)	Heart Rate Start (bpm)	Heart Rate Max (bpm)	Total Calories Burned (kcals)	Perceived Effort 1-10

Exercise Description		Set 1	Set 2	Set 3	Set 4	Set 5
	Time/Reps					
	Type/Lbs.					
	Time/Reps					
	Type/Lbs.					
	Time/Reps					
	Type/Lbs.					
	Time/Reps					
	Type/Lbs.					
	Time/Reps					
	Type/Lbs.					
	Time/Reps					
	Type/Lbs.					

Water/Fluids (oz)	Protein (grams)	Fiber (grams)	Fat (grams)	Carbs (grams)	Sugar (grams)	Sodium (grams)	Total Calories	Body Weight

Breakfast: Lunch and Snacks: Dinner:

_____   _____   _____

_____   _____   _____

_____   _____   _____

Meditation (mins)	Breathing Ex. (mins)	Sleep (hours)	Total Steps	Exercise (mins)	Flights Climbed	Standing (hours)	Stretching (mins)	Self Massage (mins)

Thoughts and Feelings:

Daily Fitness Tracker   Day 35

Did you know? Because of the endorphins released during exercise it actually gives you more energy. Also, the stamina, strength and endurance gains will keep you feeling energetic.

Date: _____ Start Time: _____ Finish Time: _____

Cardio Description	Duration (mins)	Heart Rate Start (bpm)	Heart Rate Max (bpm)	Total Calories Burned (kcals)	Perceived Effort 1-10

Exercise Description		Set 1	Set 2	Set 3	Set 4	Set 5
	Time/Reps					
	Type/Lbs.					
	Time/Reps					
	Type/Lbs.					
	Time/Reps					
	Type/Lbs.					
	Time/Reps					
	Type/Lbs.					
	Time/Reps					
	Type/Lbs.					
	Time/Reps					
	Type/Lbs.					

Water/Fluids (oz)	Protein (grams)	Fiber (grams)	Fat (grams)	Carbs (grams)	Sugar (grams)	Sodium (grams)	Total Calories	Body Weight

Breakfast: Lunch and Snacks: Dinner:

_____   _____   _____

_____   _____   _____

_____   _____   _____

Meditation (mins)	Breathing Ex. (mins)	Sleep (hours)	Total Steps	Exercise (mins)	Flights Climbed	Standing (hours)	Stretching (mins)	Self Massage (mins)

Thoughts and Feelings:

Daily Fitness Tracker   **Day 36**

"Do not let what you cannot do interfere with what you can do." – John Wooden

Date: _____ Start Time: _____ Finish Time: _____

Cardio Description	Duration (mins)	Heart Rate Start (bpm)	Heart Rate Max (bpm)	Total Calories Burned (kcals)	Perceived Effort 1-10

Exercise Description		Set 1	Set 2	Set 3	Set 4	Set 5
	Time/Reps					
	Type/Lbs.					
	Time/Reps					
	Type/Lbs.					
	Time/Reps					
	Type/Lbs.					
	Time/Reps					
	Type/Lbs.					
	Time/Reps					
	Type/Lbs.					
	Time/Reps					
	Type/Lbs.					

Water/Fluids (oz)	Protein (grams)	Fiber (grams)	Fat (grams)	Carbs (grams)	Sugar (grams)	Sodium (grams)	Total Calories	Body Weight

Breakfast: Lunch and Snacks: Dinner:

_____   _____   _____

_____   _____   _____

_____   _____   _____

Meditation (mins)	Breathing Ex. (mins)	Sleep (hours)	Total Steps	Exercise (mins)	Flights Climbed	Standing (hours)	Stretching (mins)	Self Massage (mins)

Thoughts and Feelings:

Daily Fitness Tracker   **Day 37**

"Begin with the end in mind." – Stephen Covey

Date: _____ Start Time: _____ Finish Time: _____

Cardio Description	Duration (mins)	Heart Rate Start (bpm)	Heart Rate Max (bpm)	Total Calories Burned (kcals)	Perceived Effort 1-10

Exercise Description		Set 1	Set 2	Set 3	Set 4	Set 5
	Time/Reps					
	Type/Lbs.					
	Time/Reps					
	Type/Lbs.					
	Time/Reps					
	Type/Lbs.					
	Time/Reps					
	Type/Lbs.					
	Time/Reps					
	Type/Lbs.					
	Time/Reps					
	Type/Lbs.					

Water/Fluids (oz)	Protein (grams)	Fiber (grams)	Fat (grams)	Carbs (grams)	Sugar (grams)	Sodium (grams)	Total Calories	Body Weight

Breakfast: Lunch and Snacks: Dinner:

_____   _____   _____

_____   _____   _____

_____   _____   _____

Meditation (mins)	Breathing Ex. (mins)	Sleep (hours)	Total Steps	Exercise (mins)	Flights Climbed	Standing (hours)	Stretching (mins)	Self Massage (mins)

Thoughts and Feelings:

Daily Fitness Tracker   Day 38

Did you know? Exercise may make you feel more tired at first. But over time will give you more energy and strength. The more often you take the stairs, the easier it is to take the stairs.

Date: _____ Start Time: _____ Finish Time: _____

Cardio Description	Duration (mins)	Heart Rate Start (bpm)	Heart Rate Max (bpm)	Total Calories Burned (kcals)	Perceived Effort 1-10

Exercise Description		Set 1	Set 2	Set 3	Set 4	Set 5
	Time/Reps					
	Type/Lbs.					
	Time/Reps					
	Type/Lbs.					
	Time/Reps					
	Type/Lbs.					
	Time/Reps					
	Type/Lbs.					
	Time/Reps					
	Type/Lbs.					
	Time/Reps					
	Type/Lbs.					

Water/Fluids (oz)	Protein (grams)	Fiber (grams)	Fat (grams)	Carbs (grams)	Sugar (grams)	Sodium (grams)	Total Calories	Body Weight

Breakfast: Lunch and Snacks: Dinner:

_____   _____   _____

_____   _____   _____

_____   _____   _____

Meditation (mins)	Breathing Ex. (mins)	Sleep (hours)	Total Steps	Exercise (mins)	Flights Climbed	Standing (hours)	Stretching (mins)	Self Massage (mins)

Thoughts and Feelings:

Daily Fitness Tracker   Day 39

Exercising with your children, spouse or friends can strengthen your bond with them. It is always more fun with a partner, and the endorphins will strengthen your friendship.

Date: _____ Start Time: _____ Finish Time: _____

Cardio Description	Duration (mins)	Heart Rate Start (bpm)	Heart Rate Max (bpm)	Total Calories Burned (kcals)	Perceived Effort 1-10

Exercise Description		Set 1	Set 2	Set 3	Set 4	Set 5
	Time/Reps					
	Type/Lbs.					
	Time/Reps					
	Type/Lbs.					
	Time/Reps					
	Type/Lbs.					
	Time/Reps					
	Type/Lbs.					
	Time/Reps					
	Type/Lbs.					
	Time/Reps					
	Type/Lbs.					

Water/Fluids (oz)	Protein (grams)	Fiber (grams)	Fat (grams)	Carbs (grams)	Sugar (grams)	Sodium (grams)	Total Calories	Body Weight

Breakfast: Lunch and Snacks: Dinner:

_____   _____   _____

_____   _____   _____

_____   _____   _____

Meditation (mins)	Breathing Ex. (mins)	Sleep (hours)	Total Steps	Exercise (mins)	Flights Climbed	Standing (hours)	Stretching (mins)	Self Massage (mins)

Thoughts and Feelings:

Daily Fitness Tracker   **Day 40**

Did you know? Long-term weight loss and fitness goals are much more attainable for people that have workout partners or at least some kind of social support network for reinforcement.

Date: _____ Start Time: _____ Finish Time: _____

Cardio Description	Duration (mins)	Heart Rate Start (bpm)	Heart Rate Max (bpm)	Total Calories Burned (kcals)	Perceived Effort 1-10

Exercise Description		Set 1	Set 2	Set 3	Set 4	Set 5
	Time/Reps					
	Type/Lbs.					
	Time/Reps					
	Type/Lbs.					
	Time/Reps					
	Type/Lbs.					
	Time/Reps					
	Type/Lbs.					
	Time/Reps					
	Type/Lbs.					
	Time/Reps					
	Type/Lbs.					

Water/Fluids (oz)	Protein (grams)	Fiber (grams)	Fat (grams)	Carbs (grams)	Sugar (grams)	Sodium (grams)	Total Calories	Body Weight

Breakfast: Lunch and Snacks: Dinner:

_____   _____   _____

_____   _____   _____

_____   _____   _____

Meditation (mins)	Breathing Ex. (mins)	Sleep (hours)	Total Steps	Exercise (mins)	Flights Climbed	Standing (hours)	Stretching (mins)	Self Massage (mins)

Thoughts and Feelings:

Daily Fitness Tracker   Day 41

"Believe you can and you are half way there." – Theodore Roosevelt

Date: _____ Start Time: _____ Finish Time: _____

Cardio Description	Duration (mins)	Heart Rate Start (bpm)	Heart Rate Max (bpm)	Total Calories Burned (kcals)	Perceived Effort 1-10

Exercise Description		Set 1	Set 2	Set 3	Set 4	Set 5
	Time/Reps					
	Type/Lbs.					
	Time/Reps					
	Type/Lbs.					
	Time/Reps					
	Type/Lbs.					
	Time/Reps					
	Type/Lbs.					
	Time/Reps					
	Type/Lbs.					
	Time/Reps					
	Type/Lbs.					

Water/Fluids (oz)	Protein (grams)	Fiber (grams)	Fat (grams)	Carbs (grams)	Sugar (grams)	Sodium (grams)	Total Calories	Body Weight

Breakfast: Lunch and Snacks: Dinner:

_____   _____   _____

_____   _____   _____

_____   _____   _____

Meditation (mins)	Breathing Ex. (mins)	Sleep (hours)	Total Steps	Exercise (mins)	Flights Climbed	Standing (hours)	Stretching (mins)	Self Massage (mins)

Thoughts and Feelings:

Daily Fitness Tracker   **Day 42**

"It is never too late to become what you might have been." – Anonymous

Date: _____ Start Time: _____ Finish Time: _____

Cardio Description	Duration (mins)	Heart Rate Start (bpm)	Heart Rate Max (bpm)	Total Calories Burned (kcals)	Perceived Effort 1-10

Exercise Description		Set 1	Set 2	Set 3	Set 4	Set 5
	Time/Reps					
	Type/Lbs.					
	Time/Reps					
	Type/Lbs.					
	Time/Reps					
	Type/Lbs.					
	Time/Reps					
	Type/Lbs.					
	Time/Reps					
	Type/Lbs.					
	Time/Reps					
	Type/Lbs.					

Water/Fluids (oz)	Protein (grams)	Fiber (grams)	Fat (grams)	Carbs (grams)	Sugar (grams)	Sodium (grams)	Total Calories	Body Weight

Breakfast: Lunch and Snacks: Dinner:

_____   _____   _____

_____   _____   _____

_____   _____   _____

Meditation (mins)	Breathing Ex. (mins)	Sleep (hours)	Total Steps	Exercise (mins)	Flights Climbed	Standing (hours)	Stretching (mins)	Self Massage (mins)

Thoughts and Feelings:

Daily Fitness Tracker   **Day 43**

"It takes as much energy to wish as it does to plan." – Eleanor Roosevelt

Date: _____ Start Time: _____ Finish Time: _____

Cardio Description	Duration (mins)	Heart Rate Start (bpm)	Heart Rate Max (bpm)	Total Calories Burned (kcals)	Perceived Effort 1-10

Exercise Description		Set 1	Set 2	Set 3	Set 4	Set 5
	Time/Reps					
	Type/Lbs.					
	Time/Reps					
	Type/Lbs.					
	Time/Reps					
	Type/Lbs.					
	Time/Reps					
	Type/Lbs.					
	Time/Reps					
	Type/Lbs.					
	Time/Reps					
	Type/Lbs.					

Water/Fluids (oz)	Protein (grams)	Fiber (grams)	Fat (grams)	Carbs (grams)	Sugar (grams)	Sodium (grams)	Total Calories	Body Weight

Breakfast: Lunch and Snacks: Dinner:

_____   _____   _____

_____   _____   _____

_____   _____   _____

Meditation (mins)	Breathing Ex. (mins)	Sleep (hours)	Total Steps	Exercise (mins)	Flights Climbed	Standing (hours)	Stretching (mins)	Self Massage (mins)

Thoughts and Feelings:

Daily Fitness Tracker   **Day 44**

"I don't count my sit-ups. I only start counting when it starts hurting because they're the only ones that count." – Muhammad Ali

Date: _____ Start Time: _____ Finish Time: _____

Cardio Description	Duration (mins)	Heart Rate Start (bpm)	Heart Rate Max (bpm)	Total Calories Burned (kcals)	Perceived Effort 1-10

Exercise Description		Set 1	Set 2	Set 3	Set 4	Set 5
	Time/Reps					
	Type/Lbs.					
	Time/Reps					
	Type/Lbs.					
	Time/Reps					
	Type/Lbs.					
	Time/Reps					
	Type/Lbs.					
	Time/Reps					
	Type/Lbs.					
	Time/Reps					
	Type/Lbs.					

Water/Fluids (oz)	Protein (grams)	Fiber (grams)	Fat (grams)	Carbs (grams)	Sugar (grams)	Sodium (grams)	Total Calories	Body Weight

Breakfast: Lunch and Snacks: Dinner:

_____   _____   _____

_____   _____   _____

_____   _____   _____

Meditation (mins)	Breathing Ex. (mins)	Sleep (hours)	Total Steps	Exercise (mins)	Flights Climbed	Standing (hours)	Stretching (mins)	Self Massage (mins)

Thoughts and Feelings:

Daily Fitness Tracker   Day 45

"Good things happen to those who hustle." – Anais Nin

Date: _____ Start Time: _____ Finish Time: _____

Cardio Description	Duration (mins)	Heart Rate Start (bpm)	Heart Rate Max (bpm)	Total Calories Burned (kcals)	Perceived Effort 1-10

Exercise Description		Set 1	Set 2	Set 3	Set 4	Set 5
	Time/Reps					
	Type/Lbs.					
	Time/Reps					
	Type/Lbs.					
	Time/Reps					
	Type/Lbs.					
	Time/Reps					
	Type/Lbs.					
	Time/Reps					
	Type/Lbs.					
	Time/Reps					
	Type/Lbs.					

Water/Fluids (oz)	Protein (grams)	Fiber (grams)	Fat (grams)	Carbs (grams)	Sugar (grams)	Sodium (grams)	Total Calories	Body Weight

Breakfast: Lunch and Snacks: Dinner:

_____   _____   _____

_____   _____   _____

_____   _____   _____

Meditation (mins)	Breathing Ex. (mins)	Sleep (hours)	Total Steps	Exercise (mins)	Flights Climbed	Standing (hours)	Stretching (mins)	Self Massage (mins)

Thoughts and Feelings:

Daily Fitness Tracker   **Day 46**

"Success usually comes to those who are too busy to be looking for it." – Henry David Thoreau

Date: _____ Start Time: _____ Finish Time: _____

Cardio Description	Duration (mins)	Heart Rate Start (bpm)	Heart Rate Max (bpm)	Total Calories Burned (kcals)	Perceived Effort 1-10

Exercise Description		Set 1	Set 2	Set 3	Set 4	Set 5
	Time/Reps					
	Type/Lbs.					
	Time/Reps					
	Type/Lbs.					
	Time/Reps					
	Type/Lbs.					
	Time/Reps					
	Type/Lbs.					
	Time/Reps					
	Type/Lbs.					
	Time/Reps					
	Type/Lbs.					

Water/Fluids (oz)	Protein (grams)	Fiber (grams)	Fat (grams)	Carbs (grams)	Sugar (grams)	Sodium (grams)	Total Calories	Body Weight

Breakfast: Lunch and Snacks: Dinner:

_____   _____   _____

_____   _____   _____

_____   _____   _____

Meditation (mins)	Breathing Ex. (mins)	Sleep (hours)	Total Steps	Exercise (mins)	Flights Climbed	Standing (hours)	Stretching (mins)	Self Massage (mins)

Thoughts and Feelings:

Daily Fitness Tracker   **Day 47**

"Persistence and determination alone are omnipotent. The slogan, 'Press on,' has solved and always will solve the problems of the human race." – Calvin Coolidge

Date: _____ Start Time: _____ Finish Time: _____

Cardio Description	Duration (mins)	Heart Rate Start (bpm)	Heart Rate Max (bpm)	Total Calories Burned (kcals)	Perceived Effort 1-10

Exercise Description		Set 1	Set 2	Set 3	Set 4	Set 5
	Time/Reps					
	Type/Lbs.					
	Time/Reps					
	Type/Lbs.					
	Time/Reps					
	Type/Lbs.					
	Time/Reps					
	Type/Lbs.					
	Time/Reps					
	Type/Lbs.					
	Time/Reps					
	Type/Lbs.					

Water/Fluids (oz)	Protein (grams)	Fiber (grams)	Fat (grams)	Carbs (grams)	Sugar (grams)	Sodium (grams)	Total Calories	Body Weight

Breakfast: Lunch and Snacks: Dinner:

_____   _____   _____

_____   _____   _____

_____   _____   _____

Meditation (mins)	Breathing Ex. (mins)	Sleep (hours)	Total Steps	Exercise (mins)	Flights Climbed	Standing (hours)	Stretching (mins)	Self Massage (mins)

Thoughts and Feelings:

Daily Fitness Tracker   **Day 48**

"Don't stay in bed, unless you can make money in bed." – George Burns

Date: _____ Start Time: _____ Finish Time: _____

Cardio Description	Duration (mins)	Heart Rate Start (bpm)	Heart Rate Max (bpm)	Total Calories Burned (kcals)	Perceived Effort 1-10

Exercise Description		Set 1	Set 2	Set 3	Set 4	Set 5
	Time/Reps					
	Type/Lbs.					
	Time/Reps					
	Type/Lbs.					
	Time/Reps					
	Type/Lbs.					
	Time/Reps					
	Type/Lbs.					
	Time/Reps					
	Type/Lbs.					
	Time/Reps					
	Type/Lbs.					

Water/Fluids (oz)	Protein (grams)	Fiber (grams)	Fat (grams)	Carbs (grams)	Sugar (grams)	Sodium (grams)	Total Calories	Body Weight

Breakfast: Lunch and Snacks: Dinner:

_____   _____   _____

_____   _____   _____

_____   _____   _____

Meditation (mins)	Breathing Ex. (mins)	Sleep (hours)	Total Steps	Exercise (mins)	Flights Climbed	Standing (hours)	Stretching (mins)	Self Massage (mins)

Thoughts and Feelings:

Daily Fitness Tracker   Day 49

Did you know? Regular exercise makes your heart stronger and more efficient, reducing the build up of plaque and lowering your heart rate.

Date: _____ Start Time: _____ Finish Time: _____

Cardio Description	Duration (mins)	Heart Rate Start (bpm)	Heart Rate Max (bpm)	Total Calories Burned (kcals)	Perceived Effort 1-10

Exercise Description		Set 1	Set 2	Set 3	Set 4	Set 5
	Time/Reps					
	Type/Lbs.					
	Time/Reps					
	Type/Lbs.					
	Time/Reps					
	Type/Lbs.					
	Time/Reps					
	Type/Lbs.					
	Time/Reps					
	Type/Lbs.					
	Time/Reps					
	Type/Lbs.					

Water/Fluids (oz)	Protein (grams)	Fiber (grams)	Fat (grams)	Carbs (grams)	Sugar (grams)	Sodium (grams)	Total Calories	Body Weight

Breakfast: Lunch and Snacks: Dinner:

_____   _____   _____

_____   _____   _____

_____   _____   _____

Meditation (mins)	Breathing Ex. (mins)	Sleep (hours)	Total Steps	Exercise (mins)	Flights Climbed	Standing (hours)	Stretching (mins)	Self Massage (mins)

Thoughts and Feelings:

Daily Fitness Tracker   **Day 50**

"Failure is not the opposite of success, it is part of success. Arianna Huffington

Date: _____   Start Time: _____   Finish Time: _____

Cardio Description	Duration (mins)	Heart Rate Start (bpm)	Heart Rate Max (bpm)	Total Calories Burned (kcals)	Perceived Effort 1-10

Exercise Description		Set 1	Set 2	Set 3	Set 4	Set 5
	Time/Reps					
	Type/Lbs.					
	Time/Reps					
	Type/Lbs.					
	Time/Reps					
	Type/Lbs.					
	Time/Reps					
	Type/Lbs.					
	Time/Reps					
	Type/Lbs.					
	Time/Reps					
	Type/Lbs.					

Water/Fluids (oz)	Protein (grams)	Fiber (grams)	Fat (grams)	Carbs (grams)	Sugar (grams)	Sodium (grams)	Total Calories	Body Weight

Breakfast: Lunch and Snacks: Dinner:

_____   _____   _____

_____   _____   _____

_____   _____   _____

Meditation (mins)	Breathing Ex. (mins)	Sleep (hours)	Total Steps	Exercise (mins)	Flights Climbed	Standing (hours)	Stretching (mins)	Self Massage (mins)

Thoughts and Feelings:

Daily Fitness Tracker   Day 51

"Do one thing every day that scare you." – Elanor Roosevelt

Date: _____ Start Time: _____ Finish Time: _____

Cardio Description	Duration (mins)	Heart Rate Start (bpm)	Heart Rate Max (bpm)	Total Calories Burned (kcals)	Perceived Effort 1-10

Exercise Description		Set 1	Set 2	Set 3	Set 4	Set 5
	Time/Reps					
	Type/Lbs.					
	Time/Reps					
	Type/Lbs.					
	Time/Reps					
	Type/Lbs.					
	Time/Reps					
	Type/Lbs.					
	Time/Reps					
	Type/Lbs.					
	Time/Reps					
	Type/Lbs.					

Water/Fluids (oz)	Protein (grams)	Fiber (grams)	Fat (grams)	Carbs (grams)	Sugar (grams)	Sodium (grams)	Total Calories	Body Weight

Breakfast: Lunch and Snacks: Dinner:

_____   _____   _____

_____   _____   _____

_____   _____   _____

Meditation (mins)	Breathing Ex. (mins)	Sleep (hours)	Total Steps	Exercise (mins)	Flights Climbed	Standing (hours)	Stretching (mins)	Self Massage (mins)

Thoughts and Feelings:

Daily Fitness Tracker   Day 52

"You have to exercise, or at some point you'll just break down." – Barack Obama

Date: _____ Start Time: _____ Finish Time: _____

Cardio Description	Duration (mins)	Heart Rate Start (bpm)	Heart Rate Max (bpm)	Total Calories Burned (kcals)	Perceived Effort 1-10

Exercise Description		Set 1	Set 2	Set 3	Set 4	Set 5
	Time/Reps					
	Type/Lbs.					
	Time/Reps					
	Type/Lbs.					
	Time/Reps					
	Type/Lbs.					
	Time/Reps					
	Type/Lbs.					
	Time/Reps					
	Type/Lbs.					
	Time/Reps					
	Type/Lbs.					

Water/Fluids (oz)	Protein (grams)	Fiber (grams)	Fat (grams)	Carbs (grams)	Sugar (grams)	Sodium (grams)	Total Calories	Body Weight

Breakfast: Lunch and Snacks: Dinner:

_____   _____   _____

_____   _____   _____

_____   _____   _____

Meditation (mins)	Breathing Ex. (mins)	Sleep (hours)	Total Steps	Exercise (mins)	Flights Climbed	Standing (hours)	Stretching (mins)	Self Massage (mins)

Thoughts and Feelings:

Daily Fitness Tracker   Day 53

"We are what we repeatedly do. Excellence then is not an act but a habit." – Aristotle

Date: _____ Start Time: _____ Finish Time: _____

Cardio Description	Duration (mins)	Heart Rate Start (bpm)	Heart Rate Max (bpm)	Total Calories Burned (kcals)	Perceived Effort 1-10

Exercise Description		Set 1	Set 2	Set 3	Set 4	Set 5
	Time/Reps					
	Type/Lbs.					
	Time/Reps					
	Type/Lbs.					
	Time/Reps					
	Type/Lbs.					
	Time/Reps					
	Type/Lbs.					
	Time/Reps					
	Type/Lbs.					
	Time/Reps					
	Type/Lbs.					

Water/Fluids (oz)	Protein (grams)	Fiber (grams)	Fat (grams)	Carbs (grams)	Sugar (grams)	Sodium (grams)	Total Calories	Body Weight

Breakfast: Lunch and Snacks: Dinner:

_____   _____   _____

_____   _____   _____

_____   _____   _____

Meditation (mins)	Breathing Ex. (mins)	Sleep (hours)	Total Steps	Exercise (mins)	Flights Climbed	Standing (hours)	Stretching (mins)	Self Massage (mins)

Thoughts and Feelings:

Daily Fitness Tracker   Day 54

"The true measure of a man is how he treats someone who can do him absolutely no good." –
Samuel Johnson

Date: _____ Start Time: _____ Finish Time: _____

Cardio Description	Duration (mins)	Heart Rate Start (bpm)	Heart Rate Max (bpm)	Total Calories Burned (kcals)	Perceived Effort 1-10

Exercise Description		Set 1	Set 2	Set 3	Set 4	Set 5
	Time/Reps					
	Type/Lbs.					
	Time/Reps					
	Type/Lbs.					
	Time/Reps					
	Type/Lbs.					
	Time/Reps					
	Type/Lbs.					
	Time/Reps					
	Type/Lbs.					
	Time/Reps					
	Type/Lbs.					

Water/Fluids (oz)	Protein (grams)	Fiber (grams)	Fat (grams)	Carbs (grams)	Sugar (grams)	Sodium (grams)	Total Calories	Body Weight

Breakfast: Lunch and Snacks: Dinner:

_____   _____   _____

_____   _____   _____

_____   _____   _____

Meditation (mins)	Breathing Ex. (mins)	Sleep (hours)	Total Steps	Exercise (mins)	Flights Climbed	Standing (hours)	Stretching (mins)	Self Massage (mins)

Thoughts and Feelings:

Daily Fitness Tracker   Day 55

"We never desire passionately what we desire through reason alone." – *La Rochefoucauld*

Date: _____ Start Time: _____ Finish Time: _____

Cardio Description	Duration (mins)	Heart Rate Start (bpm)	Heart Rate Max (bpm)	Total Calories Burned (kcals)	Perceived Effort 1-10

Exercise Description		Set 1	Set 2	Set 3	Set 4	Set 5
	Time/Reps					
	Type/Lbs.					
	Time/Reps					
	Type/Lbs.					
	Time/Reps					
	Type/Lbs.					
	Time/Reps					
	Type/Lbs.					
	Time/Reps					
	Type/Lbs.					
	Time/Reps					
	Type/Lbs.					

Water/Fluids (oz)	Protein (grams)	Fiber (grams)	Fat (grams)	Carbs (grams)	Sugar (grams)	Sodium (grams)	Total Calories	Body Weight

Breakfast: Lunch and Snacks: Dinner:

_____   _____   _____

_____   _____   _____

_____   _____   _____

Meditation (mins)	Breathing Ex. (mins)	Sleep (hours)	Total Steps	Exercise (mins)	Flights Climbed	Standing (hours)	Stretching (mins)	Self Massage (mins)

Thoughts and Feelings:

Daily Fitness Tracker

Day 56

"All truly great thoughts are conceived while walking." – Friedrich Nietzsche

Date: _____ Start Time: _____ Finish Time: _____

Cardio Description	Duration (mins)	Heart Rate Start (bpm)	Heart Rate Max (bpm)	Total Calories Burned (kcals)	Perceived Effort 1-10

Exercise Description		Set 1	Set 2	Set 3	Set 4	Set 5
	Time/Reps					
	Type/Lbs.					
	Time/Reps					
	Type/Lbs.					
	Time/Reps					
	Type/Lbs.					
	Time/Reps					
	Type/Lbs.					
	Time/Reps					
	Type/Lbs.					
	Time/Reps					
	Type/Lbs.					

Water/Fluids (oz)	Protein (grams)	Fiber (grams)	Fat (grams)	Carbs (grams)	Sugar (grams)	Sodium (grams)	Total Calories	Body Weight

Breakfast:

_____

_____

_____

Lunch and Snacks:

_____

_____

_____

Dinner:

_____

_____

_____

Meditation (mins)	Breathing Ex. (mins)	Sleep (hours)	Total Steps	Exercise (mins)	Flights Climbed	Standing (hours)	Stretching (mins)	Self Massage (mins)

Thoughts and Feelings:

Daily Fitness Tracker   **Day 57**

"Get comfortable with being uncomfortable." – Jillian Michaels

Date: _____ Start Time: _____ Finish Time: _____

Cardio Description	Duration (mins)	Heart Rate Start (bpm)	Heart Rate Max (bpm)	Total Calories Burned (kcals)	Perceived Effort 1-10

Exercise Description		Set 1	Set 2	Set 3	Set 4	Set 5
	Time/Reps					
	Type/Lbs.					
	Time/Reps					
	Type/Lbs.					
	Time/Reps					
	Type/Lbs.					
	Time/Reps					
	Type/Lbs.					
	Time/Reps					
	Type/Lbs.					
	Time/Reps					
	Type/Lbs.					

Water/Fluids (oz)	Protein (grams)	Fiber (grams)	Fat (grams)	Carbs (grams)	Sugar (grams)	Sodium (grams)	Total Calories	Body Weight

Breakfast: Lunch and Snacks: Dinner:

_____   _____   _____

_____   _____   _____

_____   _____   _____

Meditation (mins)	Breathing Ex. (mins)	Sleep (hours)	Total Steps	Exercise (mins)	Flights Climbed	Standing (hours)	Stretching (mins)	Self Massage (mins)

Thoughts and Feelings:

Daily Fitness Tracker   **Day 58**

"If you are in a bad mood go for a walk. If you are still in a bad mood go for another walk." – *Hippocrates*

Date: _____ Start Time: _____ Finish Time: _____

Cardio Description	Duration (mins)	Heart Rate Start (bpm)	Heart Rate Max (bpm)	Total Calories Burned (kcals)	Perceived Effort 1-10

Exercise Description		Set 1	Set 2	Set 3	Set 4	Set 5
	Time/Reps					
	Type/Lbs.					
	Time/Reps					
	Type/Lbs.					
	Time/Reps					
	Type/Lbs.					
	Time/Reps					
	Type/Lbs.					
	Time/Reps					
	Type/Lbs.					
	Time/Reps					
	Type/Lbs.					

Water/Fluids (oz)	Protein (grams)	Fiber (grams)	Fat (grams)	Carbs (grams)	Sugar (grams)	Sodium (grams)	Total Calories	Body Weight

Breakfast: Lunch and Snacks: Dinner:

_____   _____   _____

_____   _____   _____

_____   _____   _____

Meditation (mins)	Breathing Ex. (mins)	Sleep (hours)	Total Steps	Exercise (mins)	Flights Climbed	Standing (hours)	Stretching (mins)	Self Massage (mins)

Thoughts and Feelings:

Daily Fitness Tracker   **Day 59**

"If I liked food and disliked exercise as much as a 400 pound guy, I'd be a 400 pound guy." –
Scott Adams

Date: _____ Start Time: _____ Finish Time: _____

Cardio Description	Duration (mins)	Heart Rate Start (bpm)	Heart Rate Max (bpm)	Total Calories Burned (kcals)	Perceived Effort 1-10

Exercise Description		Set 1	Set 2	Set 3	Set 4	Set 5
	Time/Reps					
	Type/Lbs.					
	Time/Reps					
	Type/Lbs.					
	Time/Reps					
	Type/Lbs.					
	Time/Reps					
	Type/Lbs.					
	Time/Reps					
	Type/Lbs.					
	Time/Reps					
	Type/Lbs.					

Water/Fluids (oz)	Protein (grams)	Fiber (grams)	Fat (grams)	Carbs (grams)	Sugar (grams)	Sodium (grams)	Total Calories	Body Weight

Breakfast: Lunch and Snacks: Dinner:

_____   _____   _____

_____   _____   _____

_____   _____   _____

Meditation (mins)	Breathing Ex. (mins)	Sleep (hours)	Total Steps	Exercise (mins)	Flights Climbed	Standing (hours)	Stretching (mins)	Self Massage (mins)

Thoughts and Feelings:

Daily Fitness Tracker   **Day 60**

"If only you start eating healthy food, you will be pleasantly surprised how easy it is to lose weight." – Subodh Gupta

Date: _____ Start Time: _____ Finish Time: _____

Cardio Description	Duration (mins)	Heart Rate Start (bpm)	Heart Rate Max (bpm)	Total Calories Burned (kcals)	Perceived Effort 1-10

Exercise Description		Set 1	Set 2	Set 3	Set 4	Set 5
	Time/Reps					
	Type/Lbs.					
	Time/Reps					
	Type/Lbs.					
	Time/Reps					
	Type/Lbs.					
	Time/Reps					
	Type/Lbs.					
	Time/Reps					
	Type/Lbs.					
	Time/Reps					
	Type/Lbs.					

Water/Fluids (oz)	Protein (grams)	Fiber (grams)	Fat (grams)	Carbs (grams)	Sugar (grams)	Sodium (grams)	Total Calories	Body Weight

Breakfast: Lunch and Snacks: Dinner:

_____   _____   _____

_____   _____   _____

_____   _____   _____

Meditation (mins)	Breathing Ex. (mins)	Sleep (hours)	Total Steps	Exercise (mins)	Flights Climbed	Standing (hours)	Stretching (mins)	Self Massage (mins)

Thoughts and Feelings:

Daily Fitness Tracker   Day 61

"Not less than two hours a day should be devoted to exercise, and the weather should be little regarded." – Thomas Jefferson

Date: _____ Start Time: _____ Finish Time: _____

Cardio Description	Duration (mins)	Heart Rate Start (bpm)	Heart Rate Max (bpm)	Total Calories Burned (kcals)	Perceived Effort 1-10

Exercise Description		Set 1	Set 2	Set 3	Set 4	Set 5
	Time/Reps					
	Type/Lbs.					
	Time/Reps					
	Type/Lbs.					
	Time/Reps					
	Type/Lbs.					
	Time/Reps					
	Type/Lbs.					
	Time/Reps					
	Type/Lbs.					
	Time/Reps					
	Type/Lbs.					

Water/Fluids (oz)	Protein (grams)	Fiber (grams)	Fat (grams)	Carbs (grams)	Sugar (grams)	Sodium (grams)	Total Calories	Body Weight

Breakfast: Lunch and Snacks: Dinner:

_____   _____   _____

_____   _____   _____

_____   _____   _____

Meditation (mins)	Breathing Ex. (mins)	Sleep (hours)	Total Steps	Exercise (mins)	Flights Climbed	Standing (hours)	Stretching (mins)	Self Massage (mins)

Thoughts and Feelings:

Daily Fitness Tracker   **Day 62**

"I am not what happened to me. I am what I chose to become." – Anonymous

Date: _____ Start Time: _____ Finish Time: _____

Cardio Description	Duration (mins)	Heart Rate Start (bpm)	Heart Rate Max (bpm)	Total Calories Burned (kcals)	Perceived Effort 1-10

Exercise Description		Set 1	Set 2	Set 3	Set 4	Set 5
	Time/Reps					
	Type/Lbs.					
	Time/Reps					
	Type/Lbs.					
	Time/Reps					
	Type/Lbs.					
	Time/Reps					
	Type/Lbs.					
	Time/Reps					
	Type/Lbs.					
	Time/Reps					
	Type/Lbs.					

Water/Fluids (oz)	Protein (grams)	Fiber (grams)	Fat (grams)	Carbs (grams)	Sugar (grams)	Sodium (grams)	Total Calories	Body Weight

Breakfast: Lunch and Snacks: Dinner:

_____   _____   _____

_____   _____   _____

_____   _____   _____

Meditation (mins)	Breathing Ex. (mins)	Sleep (hours)	Total Steps	Exercise (mins)	Flights Climbed	Standing (hours)	Stretching (mins)	Self Massage (mins)

Thoughts and Feelings:

Daily Fitness Tracker

Day 63

"Goals transform a random walk into a chase." – Mihaly Csikszentmihalyi

Date: _____ Start Time: _____ Finish Time: _____

Cardio Description	Duration (mins)	Heart Rate Start (bpm)	Heart Rate Max (bpm)	Total Calories Burned (kcals)	Perceived Effort 1-10

Exercise Description		Set 1	Set 2	Set 3	Set 4	Set 5
	Time/Reps					
	Type/Lbs.					
	Time/Reps					
	Type/Lbs.					
	Time/Reps					
	Type/Lbs.					
	Time/Reps					
	Type/Lbs.					
	Time/Reps					
	Type/Lbs.					
	Time/Reps					
	Type/Lbs.					

Water/Fluids (oz)	Protein (grams)	Fiber (grams)	Fat (grams)	Carbs (grams)	Sugar (grams)	Sodium (grams)	Total Calories	Body Weight

Breakfast:

_____

_____

_____

Lunch and Snacks:

_____

_____

_____

Dinner:

_____

_____

_____

Meditation (mins)	Breathing Ex. (mins)	Sleep (hours)	Total Steps	Exercise (mins)	Flights Climbed	Standing (hours)	Stretching (mins)	Self Massage (mins)

Thoughts and Feelings:

Daily Fitness Tracker   **Day 64**

"Life is healthy, but lifestyle makes it unhealthy." – Amit Kalantri

Date: _____ Start Time: _____ Finish Time: _____

Cardio Description	Duration (mins)	Heart Rate Start (bpm)	Heart Rate Max (bpm)	Total Calories Burned (kcals)	Perceived Effort 1-10

Exercise Description		Set 1	Set 2	Set 3	Set 4	Set 5
	Time/Reps					
	Type/Lbs.					
	Time/Reps					
	Type/Lbs.					
	Time/Reps					
	Type/Lbs.					
	Time/Reps					
	Type/Lbs.					
	Time/Reps					
	Type/Lbs.					
	Time/Reps					
	Type/Lbs.					

Water/Fluids (oz)	Protein (grams)	Fiber (grams)	Fat (grams)	Carbs (grams)	Sugar (grams)	Sodium (grams)	Total Calories	Body Weight

Breakfast: Lunch and Snacks: Dinner:

_____   _____   _____

_____   _____   _____

_____   _____   _____

Meditation (mins)	Breathing Ex. (mins)	Sleep (hours)	Total Steps	Exercise (mins)	Flights Climbed	Standing (hours)	Stretching (mins)	Self Massage (mins)

Thoughts and Feelings:

Daily Fitness Tracker   **Day 65**

"When we are active, we become stronger and more energetic. This, in turn, makes us more positive and self-confident. It's a powerful cycle." – Ernest Cadorin

Date: _____ Start Time: _____ Finish Time: _____

Cardio Description	Duration (mins)	Heart Rate Start (bpm)	Heart Rate Max (bpm)	Total Calories Burned (kcals)	Perceived Effort 1-10

Exercise Description		Set 1	Set 2	Set 3	Set 4	Set 5
	Time/Reps					
	Type/Lbs.					
	Time/Reps					
	Type/Lbs.					
	Time/Reps					
	Type/Lbs.					
	Time/Reps					
	Type/Lbs.					
	Time/Reps					
	Type/Lbs.					
	Time/Reps					
	Type/Lbs.					

Water/Fluids (oz)	Protein (grams)	Fiber (grams)	Fat (grams)	Carbs (grams)	Sugar (grams)	Sodium (grams)	Total Calories	Body Weight

Breakfast: Lunch and Snacks: Dinner:

_____   _____   _____

_____   _____   _____

_____   _____   _____

Meditation (mins)	Breathing Ex. (mins)	Sleep (hours)	Total Steps	Exercise (mins)	Flights Climbed	Standing (hours)	Stretching (mins)	Self Massage (mins)

Thoughts and Feelings:

Daily Fitness Tracker   Day 66

*"Most people stop eating not when their stomachs are full but when their plates are empty." –
Mokokoma Mokhonoana*

Date: _____ Start Time: _____ Finish Time: _____

Cardio Description	Duration (mins)	Heart Rate Start (bpm)	Heart Rate Max (bpm)	Total Calories Burned (kcals)	Perceived Effort 1-10

Exercise Description		Set 1	Set 2	Set 3	Set 4	Set 5
	Time/Reps					
	Type/Lbs.					
	Time/Reps					
	Type/Lbs.					
	Time/Reps					
	Type/Lbs.					
	Time/Reps					
	Type/Lbs.					
	Time/Reps					
	Type/Lbs.					
	Time/Reps					
	Type/Lbs.					

Water/Fluids (oz)	Protein (grams)	Fiber (grams)	Fat (grams)	Carbs (grams)	Sugar (grams)	Sodium (grams)	Total Calories	Body Weight

Breakfast: Lunch and Snacks: Dinner:

_____   _____   _____
_____   _____   _____
_____   _____   _____

Meditation (mins)	Breathing Ex. (mins)	Sleep (hours)	Total Steps	Exercise (mins)	Flights Climbed	Standing (hours)	Stretching (mins)	Self Massage (mins)

Thoughts and Feelings:

Daily Fitness Tracker   **Day 67**

"Run likes you're chasing somebody who owes you money." – Toni Sorenson

Date: _____ Start Time: _____ Finish Time: _____

Cardio Description	Duration (mins)	Heart Rate Start (bpm)	Heart Rate Max (bpm)	Total Calories Burned (kcals)	Perceived Effort 1-10

Exercise Description		Set 1	Set 2	Set 3	Set 4	Set 5
	Time/Reps					
	Type/Lbs.					
	Time/Reps					
	Type/Lbs.					
	Time/Reps					
	Type/Lbs.					
	Time/Reps					
	Type/Lbs.					
	Time/Reps					
	Type/Lbs.					
	Time/Reps					
	Type/Lbs.					

Water/Fluids (oz)	Protein (grams)	Fiber (grams)	Fat (grams)	Carbs (grams)	Sugar (grams)	Sodium (grams)	Total Calories	Body Weight

Breakfast: Lunch and Snacks: Dinner:

_____   _____   _____

_____   _____   _____

_____   _____   _____

Meditation (mins)	Breathing Ex. (mins)	Sleep (hours)	Total Steps	Exercise (mins)	Flights Climbed	Standing (hours)	Stretching (mins)	Self Massage (mins)

Thoughts and Feelings:

Daily Fitness Tracker   **Day 68**

"The reason I exercise is for the quality of life I enjoy." – Kenneth H. Cooper

Date: _____ Start Time: _____ Finish Time: _____

Cardio Description	Duration (mins)	Heart Rate Start (bpm)	Heart Rate Max (bpm)	Total Calories Burned (kcals)	Perceived Effort 1-10

Exercise Description		Set 1	Set 2	Set 3	Set 4	Set 5
	Time/Reps					
	Type/Lbs.					
	Time/Reps					
	Type/Lbs.					
	Time/Reps					
	Type/Lbs.					
	Time/Reps					
	Type/Lbs.					
	Time/Reps					
	Type/Lbs.					
	Time/Reps					
	Type/Lbs.					

Water/Fluids (oz)	Protein (grams)	Fiber (grams)	Fat (grams)	Carbs (grams)	Sugar (grams)	Sodium (grams)	Total Calories	Body Weight

Breakfast: Lunch and Snacks: Dinner:

_____   _____   _____

_____   _____   _____

_____   _____   _____

Meditation (mins)	Breathing Ex. (mins)	Sleep (hours)	Total Steps	Exercise (mins)	Flights Climbed	Standing (hours)	Stretching (mins)	Self Massage (mins)

Thoughts and Feelings:

Daily Fitness Tracker   **Day 69**

"It is not how fast or how far, but how often you run that makes you a real runner." – Toni Sorenson

Date: _____ Start Time: _____ Finish Time: _____

Cardio Description	Duration (mins)	Heart Rate Start (bpm)	Heart Rate Max (bpm)	Total Calories Burned (kcals)	Perceived Effort 1-10

Exercise Description		Set 1	Set 2	Set 3	Set 4	Set 5
	Time/Reps					
	Type/Lbs.					
	Time/Reps					
	Type/Lbs.					
	Time/Reps					
	Type/Lbs.					
	Time/Reps					
	Type/Lbs.					
	Time/Reps					
	Type/Lbs.					
	Time/Reps					
	Type/Lbs.					

Water/Fluids (oz)	Protein (grams)	Fiber (grams)	Fat (grams)	Carbs (grams)	Sugar (grams)	Sodium (grams)	Total Calories	Body Weight

Breakfast: Lunch and Snacks: Dinner:

_____   _____   _____

_____   _____   _____

_____   _____   _____

Meditation (mins)	Breathing Ex. (mins)	Sleep (hours)	Total Steps	Exercise (mins)	Flights Climbed	Standing (hours)	Stretching (mins)	Self Massage (mins)

Thoughts and Feelings:

Daily Fitness Tracker   Day 70

Did you know? Your body not only needs movement, but also varied movement. To get oxygen and nutrients to your tissues you have to move in ways that you are not used to moving.

Date: _____ Start Time: _____ Finish Time: _____

Cardio Description	Duration (mins)	Heart Rate Start (bpm)	Heart Rate Max (bpm)	Total Calories Burned (kcals)	Perceived Effort 1-10

Exercise Description		Set 1	Set 2	Set 3	Set 4	Set 5
	Time/Reps					
	Type/Lbs.					
	Time/Reps					
	Type/Lbs.					
	Time/Reps					
	Type/Lbs.					
	Time/Reps					
	Type/Lbs.					
	Time/Reps					
	Type/Lbs.					
	Time/Reps					
	Type/Lbs.					

Water/Fluids (oz)	Protein (grams)	Fiber (grams)	Fat (grams)	Carbs (grams)	Sugar (grams)	Sodium (grams)	Total Calories	Body Weight

Breakfast: Lunch and Snacks: Dinner:

_____   _____   _____

_____   _____   _____

_____   _____   _____

Meditation (mins)	Breathing Ex. (mins)	Sleep (hours)	Total Steps	Exercise (mins)	Flights Climbed	Standing (hours)	Stretching (mins)	Self Massage (mins)

Thoughts and Feelings:

Daily Fitness Tracker   **Day 71**

Did you know? Very high intensity, low variety, repetitious exercise takes a toll. You want consistent, high variety exercise so your body can recover, heal and come back for more.

Date: _____ Start Time: _____ Finish Time: _____

Cardio Description	Duration (mins)	Heart Rate Start (bpm)	Heart Rate Max (bpm)	Total Calories Burned (kcals)	Perceived Effort 1-10

Exercise Description		Set 1	Set 2	Set 3	Set 4	Set 5
	Time/Reps					
	Type/Lbs.					
	Time/Reps					
	Type/Lbs.					
	Time/Reps					
	Type/Lbs.					
	Time/Reps					
	Type/Lbs.					
	Time/Reps					
	Type/Lbs.					
	Time/Reps					
	Type/Lbs.					

Water/Fluids (oz)	Protein (grams)	Fiber (grams)	Fat (grams)	Carbs (grams)	Sugar (grams)	Sodium (grams)	Total Calories	Body Weight

Breakfast: Lunch and Snacks: Dinner:

_____   _____   _____

_____   _____   _____

_____   _____   _____

Meditation (mins)	Breathing Ex. (mins)	Sleep (hours)	Total Steps	Exercise (mins)	Flights Climbed	Standing (hours)	Stretching (mins)	Self Massage (mins)

Thoughts and Feelings:

Daily Fitness Tracker   **Day 72**

Your body amounts to a cellular story that you are writing every second of every day. With this in mind, write the best story you can.

Date: _____ Start Time: _____ Finish Time: _____

Cardio Description	Duration (mins)	Heart Rate Start (bpm)	Heart Rate Max (bpm)	Total Calories Burned (kcals)	Perceived Effort 1-10

Exercise Description		Set 1	Set 2	Set 3	Set 4	Set 5
	Time/Reps					
	Type/Lbs.					
	Time/Reps					
	Type/Lbs.					
	Time/Reps					
	Type/Lbs.					
	Time/Reps					
	Type/Lbs.					
	Time/Reps					
	Type/Lbs.					
	Time/Reps					
	Type/Lbs.					

Water/Fluids (oz)	Protein (grams)	Fiber (grams)	Fat (grams)	Carbs (grams)	Sugar (grams)	Sodium (grams)	Total Calories	Body Weight

Breakfast: Lunch and Snacks: Dinner:

_____   _____   _____

_____   _____   _____

_____   _____   _____

Meditation (mins)	Breathing Ex. (mins)	Sleep (hours)	Total Steps	Exercise (mins)	Flights Climbed	Standing (hours)	Stretching (mins)	Self Massage (mins)

Thoughts and Feelings:

Daily Fitness Tracker   Day 73

Cross training is necessary. Take part in as many different forms of exercise as you can so that you can bridge the gaps between the activities you partake in and those that you don't.

Date: _____ Start Time: _____ Finish Time: _____

Cardio Description	Duration (mins)	Heart Rate Start (bpm)	Heart Rate Max (bpm)	Total Calories Burned (kcals)	Perceived Effort 1-10

Exercise Description		Set 1	Set 2	Set 3	Set 4	Set 5
	Time/Reps					
	Type/Lbs.					
	Time/Reps					
	Type/Lbs.					
	Time/Reps					
	Type/Lbs.					
	Time/Reps					
	Type/Lbs.					
	Time/Reps					
	Type/Lbs.					
	Time/Reps					
	Type/Lbs.					

Water/Fluids (oz)	Protein (grams)	Fiber (grams)	Fat (grams)	Carbs (grams)	Sugar (grams)	Sodium (grams)	Total Calories	Body Weight

Breakfast: Lunch and Snacks: Dinner:

_____   _____   _____

_____   _____   _____

_____   _____   _____

Meditation (mins)	Breathing Ex. (mins)	Sleep (hours)	Total Steps	Exercise (mins)	Flights Climbed	Standing (hours)	Stretching (mins)	Self Massage (mins)

Thoughts and Feelings:

Daily Fitness Tracker   Day 74

Our bodies are capable of thousands of different physical positions and postures that we never use. Try using new positions so that you can reclaim strength and stability in those areas.

Date: _____ Start Time: _____ Finish Time: _____

Cardio Description	Duration (mins)	Heart Rate Start (bpm)	Heart Rate Max (bpm)	Total Calories Burned (kcals)	Perceived Effort 1-10

Exercise Description		Set 1	Set 2	Set 3	Set 4	Set 5
	Time/Reps					
	Type/Lbs.					
	Time/Reps					
	Type/Lbs.					
	Time/Reps					
	Type/Lbs.					
	Time/Reps					
	Type/Lbs.					
	Time/Reps					
	Type/Lbs.					
	Time/Reps					
	Type/Lbs.					

Water/Fluids (oz)	Protein (grams)	Fiber (grams)	Fat (grams)	Carbs (grams)	Sugar (grams)	Sodium (grams)	Total Calories	Body Weight

Breakfast: Lunch and Snacks: Dinner:

_____   _____   _____

_____   _____   _____

_____   _____   _____

Meditation (mins)	Breathing Ex. (mins)	Sleep (hours)	Total Steps	Exercise (mins)	Flights Climbed	Standing (hours)	Stretching (mins)	Self Massage (mins)

Thoughts and Feelings:

Daily Fitness Tracker   Day 75

Every unfamiliar joint position you can find produces a new load on tissues that are unused and atrophied.

Date: _____ Start Time: _____ Finish Time: _____

Cardio Description	Duration (mins)	Heart Rate Start (bpm)	Heart Rate Max (bpm)	Total Calories Burned (kcals)	Perceived Effort 1-10

Exercise Description		Set 1	Set 2	Set 3	Set 4	Set 5
	Time/Reps					
	Type/Lbs.					
	Time/Reps					
	Type/Lbs.					
	Time/Reps					
	Type/Lbs.					
	Time/Reps					
	Type/Lbs.					
	Time/Reps					
	Type/Lbs.					
	Time/Reps					
	Type/Lbs.					

Water/Fluids (oz)	Protein (grams)	Fiber (grams)	Fat (grams)	Carbs (grams)	Sugar (grams)	Sodium (grams)	Total Calories	Body Weight

Breakfast: Lunch and Snacks: Dinner:

_____   _____   _____

_____   _____   _____

_____   _____   _____

Meditation (mins)	Breathing Ex. (mins)	Sleep (hours)	Total Steps	Exercise (mins)	Flights Climbed	Standing (hours)	Stretching (mins)	Self Massage (mins)

Thoughts and Feelings:

Daily Fitness Tracker   Day 76

"Life can be frustrating sometimes. Take a nap, exercise, meditate or do whatever it takes to 'reboot' your thinking. Happiness is just a thought away." – Tom Giaquinto

Date: _____ Start Time: _____ Finish Time: _____

Cardio Description	Duration (mins)	Heart Rate Start (bpm)	Heart Rate Max (bpm)	Total Calories Burned (kcals)	Perceived Effort 1-10

Exercise Description		Set 1	Set 2	Set 3	Set 4	Set 5
	Time/Reps					
	Type/Lbs.					
	Time/Reps					
	Type/Lbs.					
	Time/Reps					
	Type/Lbs.					
	Time/Reps					
	Type/Lbs.					
	Time/Reps					
	Type/Lbs.					
	Time/Reps					
	Type/Lbs.					

Water/Fluids (oz)	Protein (grams)	Fiber (grams)	Fat (grams)	Carbs (grams)	Sugar (grams)	Sodium (grams)	Total Calories	Body Weight

Breakfast: Lunch and Snacks: Dinner:

_____   _____   _____

_____   _____   _____

_____   _____   _____

Meditation (mins)	Breathing Ex. (mins)	Sleep (hours)	Total Steps	Exercise (mins)	Flights Climbed	Standing (hours)	Stretching (mins)	Self Massage (mins)

Thoughts and Feelings:

Daily Fitness Tracker   Day 77

"Exercise should be regarded as tribute to the heart." – Gene Tunney

Date: _____ Start Time: _____ Finish Time: _____

Cardio Description	Duration (mins)	Heart Rate Start (bpm)	Heart Rate Max (bpm)	Total Calories Burned (kcals)	Perceived Effort 1-10

Exercise Description		Set 1	Set 2	Set 3	Set 4	Set 5
	Time/Reps					
	Type/Lbs.					
	Time/Reps					
	Type/Lbs.					
	Time/Reps					
	Type/Lbs.					
	Time/Reps					
	Type/Lbs.					
	Time/Reps					
	Type/Lbs.					
	Time/Reps					
	Type/Lbs.					

Water/Fluids (oz)	Protein (grams)	Fiber (grams)	Fat (grams)	Carbs (grams)	Sugar (grams)	Sodium (grams)	Total Calories	Body Weight

Breakfast: Lunch and Snacks: Dinner:

_____   _____   _____

_____   _____   _____

_____   _____   _____

Meditation (mins)	Breathing Ex. (mins)	Sleep (hours)	Total Steps	Exercise (mins)	Flights Climbed	Standing (hours)	Stretching (mins)	Self Massage (mins)

Thoughts and Feelings:

Daily Fitness Tracker   **Day 78**

"Practice puts brains in your muscles." – Sam Snead

Date: _____ Start Time: _____ Finish Time: _____

Cardio Description	Duration (mins)	Heart Rate Start (bpm)	Heart Rate Max (bpm)	Total Calories Burned (kcals)	Perceived Effort 1-10

Exercise Description		Set 1	Set 2	Set 3	Set 4	Set 5
	Time/Reps					
	Type/Lbs.					
	Time/Reps					
	Type/Lbs.					
	Time/Reps					
	Type/Lbs.					
	Time/Reps					
	Type/Lbs.					
	Time/Reps					
	Type/Lbs.					
	Time/Reps					
	Type/Lbs.					

Water/Fluids (oz)	Protein (grams)	Fiber (grams)	Fat (grams)	Carbs (grams)	Sugar (grams)	Sodium (grams)	Total Calories	Body Weight

Breakfast:

_____

_____

_____

Lunch and Snacks:

_____

_____

_____

Dinner:

_____

_____

_____

Meditation (mins)	Breathing Ex. (mins)	Sleep (hours)	Total Steps	Exercise (mins)	Flights Climbed	Standing (hours)	Stretching (mins)	Self Massage (mins)

Thoughts and Feelings:

Daily Fitness Tracker   **Day 79**

"Leave all afternoon for exercise and recreation, which are as necessary as reading. I will rather say more necessary because health is worth more than learning." – Thomas Jefferson

Date: _____ Start Time: _____ Finish Time: _____

Cardio Description	Duration (mins)	Heart Rate Start (bpm)	Heart Rate Max (bpm)	Total Calories Burned (kcals)	Perceived Effort 1-10

Exercise Description		Set 1	Set 2	Set 3	Set 4	Set 5
	Time/Reps					
	Type/Lbs.					
	Time/Reps					
	Type/Lbs.					
	Time/Reps					
	Type/Lbs.					
	Time/Reps					
	Type/Lbs.					
	Time/Reps					
	Type/Lbs.					
	Time/Reps					
	Type/Lbs.					

Water/Fluids (oz)	Protein (grams)	Fiber (grams)	Fat (grams)	Carbs (grams)	Sugar (grams)	Sodium (grams)	Total Calories	Body Weight

Breakfast: Lunch and Snacks: Dinner:

_____   _____   _____

_____   _____   _____

_____   _____   _____

Meditation (mins)	Breathing Ex. (mins)	Sleep (hours)	Total Steps	Exercise (mins)	Flights Climbed	Standing (hours)	Stretching (mins)	Self Massage (mins)

Thoughts and Feelings:

Daily Fitness Tracker   **Day 80**

"Fitness has nothing to do with age." – Virender Sehwag

Date: _____ Start Time: _____ Finish Time: _____

Cardio Description	Duration (mins)	Heart Rate Start (bpm)	Heart Rate Max (bpm)	Total Calories Burned (kcals)	Perceived Effort 1-10

Exercise Description		Set 1	Set 2	Set 3	Set 4	Set 5
	Time/Reps					
	Type/Lbs.					
	Time/Reps					
	Type/Lbs.					
	Time/Reps					
	Type/Lbs.					
	Time/Reps					
	Type/Lbs.					
	Time/Reps					
	Type/Lbs.					
	Time/Reps					
	Type/Lbs.					

Water/Fluids (oz)	Protein (grams)	Fiber (grams)	Fat (grams)	Carbs (grams)	Sugar (grams)	Sodium (grams)	Total Calories	Body Weight

Breakfast: Lunch and Snacks: Dinner:

_____   _____   _____

_____   _____   _____

_____   _____   _____

Meditation (mins)	Breathing Ex. (mins)	Sleep (hours)	Total Steps	Exercise (mins)	Flights Climbed	Standing (hours)	Stretching (mins)	Self Massage (mins)

Thoughts and Feelings:

Daily Fitness Tracker   Day 81

"You can be the most beautiful person on Earth, and if you don't have a fitness of diet routine, you won't be beautiful." – Martha Stewart

Date: _____ Start Time: _____ Finish Time: _____

Cardio Description	Duration (mins)	Heart Rate Start (bpm)	Heart Rate Max (bpm)	Total Calories Burned (kcals)	Perceived Effort 1-10

Exercise Description		Set 1	Set 2	Set 3	Set 4	Set 5
	Time/Reps					
	Type/Lbs.					
	Time/Reps					
	Type/Lbs.					
	Time/Reps					
	Type/Lbs.					
	Time/Reps					
	Type/Lbs.					
	Time/Reps					
	Type/Lbs.					
	Time/Reps					
	Type/Lbs.					

Water/Fluids (oz)	Protein (grams)	Fiber (grams)	Fat (grams)	Carbs (grams)	Sugar (grams)	Sodium (grams)	Total Calories	Body Weight

Breakfast: Lunch and Snacks: Dinner:

_____   _____   _____

_____   _____   _____

_____   _____   _____

Meditation (mins)	Breathing Ex. (mins)	Sleep (hours)	Total Steps	Exercise (mins)	Flights Climbed	Standing (hours)	Stretching (mins)	Self Massage (mins)

Thoughts and Feelings:

Daily Fitness Tracker   Day 82

"If a man achieves victory over this body, who in the world can exercise power over him? He who rules himself rules over the whole world." – Vinoba Bhave

Date: _____ Start Time: _____ Finish Time: _____

Cardio Description	Duration (mins)	Heart Rate Start (bpm)	Heart Rate Max (bpm)	Total Calories Burned (kcals)	Perceived Effort 1-10

Exercise Description		Set 1	Set 2	Set 3	Set 4	Set 5
	Time/Reps					
	Type/Lbs.					
	Time/Reps					
	Type/Lbs.					
	Time/Reps					
	Type/Lbs.					
	Time/Reps					
	Type/Lbs.					
	Time/Reps					
	Type/Lbs.					
	Time/Reps					
	Type/Lbs.					

Water/Fluids (oz)	Protein (grams)	Fiber (grams)	Fat (grams)	Carbs (grams)	Sugar (grams)	Sodium (grams)	Total Calories	Body Weight

Breakfast: Lunch and Snacks: Dinner:

_____   _____   _____

_____   _____   _____

_____   _____   _____

Meditation (mins)	Breathing Ex. (mins)	Sleep (hours)	Total Steps	Exercise (mins)	Flights Climbed	Standing (hours)	Stretching (mins)	Self Massage (mins)

Thoughts and Feelings:

Daily Fitness Tracker   Day 83

"You can't be fat and fast too; so lift, run, diet and work." – Hank Stram

Date: _____ Start Time: _____ Finish Time: _____

Cardio Description	Duration (mins)	Heart Rate Start (bpm)	Heart Rate Max (bpm)	Total Calories Burned (kcals)	Perceived Effort 1-10

Exercise Description		Set 1	Set 2	Set 3	Set 4	Set 5
	Time/Reps					
	Type/Lbs.					
	Time/Reps					
	Type/Lbs.					
	Time/Reps					
	Type/Lbs.					
	Time/Reps					
	Type/Lbs.					
	Time/Reps					
	Type/Lbs.					
	Time/Reps					
	Type/Lbs.					

Water/Fluids (oz)	Protein (grams)	Fiber (grams)	Fat (grams)	Carbs (grams)	Sugar (grams)	Sodium (grams)	Total Calories	Body Weight

Breakfast: Lunch and Snacks: Dinner:

_____   _____   _____

_____   _____   _____

_____   _____   _____

Meditation (mins)	Breathing Ex. (mins)	Sleep (hours)	Total Steps	Exercise (mins)	Flights Climbed	Standing (hours)	Stretching (mins)	Self Massage (mins)

Thoughts and Feelings:

Daily Fitness Tracker   Day 84

"The only way for a rich man to be healthy is by exercise and abstinence, to live as if he were poor." – William Temple

Date: _____ Start Time: _____ Finish Time: _____

Cardio Description	Duration (mins)	Heart Rate Start (bpm)	Heart Rate Max (bpm)	Total Calories Burned (kcals)	Perceived Effort 1-10

Exercise Description		Set 1	Set 2	Set 3	Set 4	Set 5
	Time/Reps					
	Type/Lbs.					
	Time/Reps					
	Type/Lbs.					
	Time/Reps					
	Type/Lbs.					
	Time/Reps					
	Type/Lbs.					
	Time/Reps					
	Type/Lbs.					
	Time/Reps					
	Type/Lbs.					

Water/Fluids (oz)	Protein (grams)	Fiber (grams)	Fat (grams)	Carbs (grams)	Sugar (grams)	Sodium (grams)	Total Calories	Body Weight

Breakfast: Lunch and Snacks: Dinner:

_____   _____   _____

_____   _____   _____

_____   _____   _____

Meditation (mins)	Breathing Ex. (mins)	Sleep (hours)	Total Steps	Exercise (mins)	Flights Climbed	Standing (hours)	Stretching (mins)	Self Massage (mins)

Thoughts and Feelings:

Daily Fitness Tracker   **Day 85**

"The best way to predict the future is to create it." – Abraham Lincoln

Date: _____ Start Time: _____ Finish Time: _____

Cardio Description	Duration (mins)	Heart Rate Start (bpm)	Heart Rate Max (bpm)	Total Calories Burned (kcals)	Perceived Effort 1-10

Exercise Description		Set 1	Set 2	Set 3	Set 4	Set 5
	Time/Reps					
	Type/Lbs.					
	Time/Reps					
	Type/Lbs.					
	Time/Reps					
	Type/Lbs.					
	Time/Reps					
	Type/Lbs.					
	Time/Reps					
	Type/Lbs.					
	Time/Reps					
	Type/Lbs.					

Water/Fluids (oz)	Protein (grams)	Fiber (grams)	Fat (grams)	Carbs (grams)	Sugar (grams)	Sodium (grams)	Total Calories	Body Weight

Breakfast: Lunch and Snacks: Dinner:

_____   _____   _____

_____   _____   _____

_____   _____   _____

Meditation (mins)	Breathing Ex. (mins)	Sleep (hours)	Total Steps	Exercise (mins)	Flights Climbed	Standing (hours)	Stretching (mins)	Self Massage (mins)

Thoughts and Feelings:

Daily Fitness Tracker   **Day 86**

Work for continual progress not immediate perfection.

Date: _____ Start Time: _____ Finish Time: _____

Cardio Description	Duration (mins)	Heart Rate Start (bpm)	Heart Rate Max (bpm)	Total Calories Burned (kcals)	Perceived Effort 1-10

Exercise Description		Set 1	Set 2	Set 3	Set 4	Set 5
	Time/Reps					
	Type/Lbs.					
	Time/Reps					
	Type/Lbs.					
	Time/Reps					
	Type/Lbs.					
	Time/Reps					
	Type/Lbs.					
	Time/Reps					
	Type/Lbs.					
	Time/Reps					
	Type/Lbs.					

Water/Fluids (oz)	Protein (grams)	Fiber (grams)	Fat (grams)	Carbs (grams)	Sugar (grams)	Sodium (grams)	Total Calories	Body Weight

Breakfast: Lunch and Snacks: Dinner:

_____   _____   _____

_____   _____   _____

_____   _____   _____

Meditation (mins)	Breathing Ex. (mins)	Sleep (hours)	Total Steps	Exercise (mins)	Flights Climbed	Standing (hours)	Stretching (mins)	Self Massage (mins)

Thoughts and Feelings:

Daily Fitness Tracker   **Day 87**

Use exercise to find joy, not to make up for the calories that you consumed.

Date: _____ Start Time: _____ Finish Time: _____

Cardio Description	Duration (mins)	Heart Rate Start (bpm)	Heart Rate Max (bpm)	Total Calories Burned (kcals)	Perceived Effort 1-10

Exercise Description		Set 1	Set 2	Set 3	Set 4	Set 5
	Time/Reps					
	Type/Lbs.					
	Time/Reps					
	Type/Lbs.					
	Time/Reps					
	Type/Lbs.					
	Time/Reps					
	Type/Lbs.					
	Time/Reps					
	Type/Lbs.					
	Time/Reps					
	Type/Lbs.					

Water/Fluids (oz)	Protein (grams)	Fiber (grams)	Fat (grams)	Carbs (grams)	Sugar (grams)	Sodium (grams)	Total Calories	Body Weight

Breakfast: Lunch and Snacks: Dinner:

_____   _____   _____

_____   _____   _____

_____   _____   _____

Meditation (mins)	Breathing Ex. (mins)	Sleep (hours)	Total Steps	Exercise (mins)	Flights Climbed	Standing (hours)	Stretching (mins)	Self Massage (mins)

Thoughts and Feelings:

Daily Fitness Tracker   **Day 88**

Going from bed, to your car, to your desk, to a booth, to a car, to the couch, and back to bed is chronic immobilization. Don't engineer physical activity out of your daily routine.

Date: _____ Start Time: _____ Finish Time: _____

Cardio Description	Duration (mins)	Heart Rate Start (bpm)	Heart Rate Max (bpm)	Total Calories Burned (kcals)	Perceived Effort 1-10

Exercise Description		Set 1	Set 2	Set 3	Set 4	Set 5
	Time/Reps					
	Type/Lbs.					
	Time/Reps					
	Type/Lbs.					
	Time/Reps					
	Type/Lbs.					
	Time/Reps					
	Type/Lbs.					
	Time/Reps					
	Type/Lbs.					
	Time/Reps					
	Type/Lbs.					

Water/Fluids (oz)	Protein (grams)	Fiber (grams)	Fat (grams)	Carbs (grams)	Sugar (grams)	Sodium (grams)	Total Calories	Body Weight

Breakfast: Lunch and Snacks: Dinner:

_____   _____   _____

_____   _____   _____

_____   _____   _____

Meditation (mins)	Breathing Ex. (mins)	Sleep (hours)	Total Steps	Exercise (mins)	Flights Climbed	Standing (hours)	Stretching (mins)	Self Massage (mins)

Thoughts and Feelings:

Daily Fitness Tracker   **Day 89**

Most humans live their lives like animals in captivity. You may not realize it, but your body knows that your routine keeps it in a confined cage. Let it out through playful exercise.

Date: _____ Start Time: _____ Finish Time: _____

Cardio Description	Duration (mins)	Heart Rate Start (bpm)	Heart Rate Max (bpm)	Total Calories Burned (kcals)	Perceived Effort 1-10

Exercise Description		Set 1	Set 2	Set 3	Set 4	Set 5
	Time/Reps					
	Type/Lbs.					
	Time/Reps					
	Type/Lbs.					
	Time/Reps					
	Type/Lbs.					
	Time/Reps					
	Type/Lbs.					
	Time/Reps					
	Type/Lbs.					
	Time/Reps					
	Type/Lbs.					

Water/Fluids (oz)	Protein (grams)	Fiber (grams)	Fat (grams)	Carbs (grams)	Sugar (grams)	Sodium (grams)	Total Calories	Body Weight

Breakfast: Lunch and Snacks: Dinner:

_____   _____   _____

_____   _____   _____

_____   _____   _____

Meditation (mins)	Breathing Ex. (mins)	Sleep (hours)	Total Steps	Exercise (mins)	Flights Climbed	Standing (hours)	Stretching (mins)	Self Massage (mins)

Thoughts and Feelings:

Daily Fitness Tracker   **Day 90**

The paleodiet is eating what our hunter gatherer ancestors would have eaten. The paleo exercise plan is constant, varied movement that both challenges and refreshes the body.

Date: _____ Start Time: _____ Finish Time: _____

Cardio Description	Duration (mins)	Heart Rate Start (bpm)	Heart Rate Max (bpm)	Total Calories Burned (kcals)	Perceived Effort 1-10

Exercise Description		Set 1	Set 2	Set 3	Set 4	Set 5
	Time/Reps					
	Type/Lbs.					
	Time/Reps					
	Type/Lbs.					
	Time/Reps					
	Type/Lbs.					
	Time/Reps					
	Type/Lbs.					
	Time/Reps					
	Type/Lbs.					
	Time/Reps					
	Type/Lbs.					

Water/Fluids (oz)	Protein (grams)	Fiber (grams)	Fat (grams)	Carbs (grams)	Sugar (grams)	Sodium (grams)	Total Calories	Body Weight

Breakfast: Lunch and Snacks: Dinner:

_____   _____   _____

_____   _____   _____

_____   _____   _____

Meditation (mins)	Breathing Ex. (mins)	Sleep (hours)	Total Steps	Exercise (mins)	Flights Climbed	Standing (hours)	Stretching (mins)	Self Massage (mins)

Thoughts and Feelings:

Visit www.programpeace.com for Much More

I would like to encourage you to get the companion book, or visit the companion website at www.programpeace.com. Here you can find hundreds of additional self-care exercises to help you reprogram your biology for health, happiness, and stress resilience. The techniques are based on a new synthesis of diverse fields, and are heavily informed by scientific facts. Use them to find the ideal postural configuration for each part of your body, extinguish the inferiority instinct, and find peace through neuroplasticity.

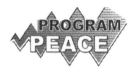

Self-Care System
Reprogram Your Brain and Body
Through Neuroplasticity

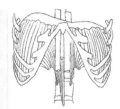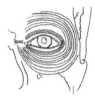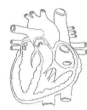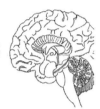

Home

About

1. Submissive Nonverbals

2. Stress Adaptation

3. Breathing Retraining

4. Eye Posture

5. Tension and Relaxation

6. Massage and Compression

7. Thinking Peacefully

8. Facial Restructuring

9. Facial Massage

Programming Yourself for Peace

Program Peace is a self-care system that will guide you to use over 100 different exercises to train your body to function optimally. Many different systems throughout the body perform suboptimally because their actions have been linked to stress, strain, and negative emotions. Over time this results in the accumulation of trauma within the body's tissues. The activities on this website can help you rehabilitate them, reducing stress, and freeing you from pain. By using this system you will experience improved posture, more energy, increased confidence, and the ability to breathe freely. The entire program is available to you on this website at no cost. Use the menu to the left to access the various exercises by "chapter" title. Each chapter addresses a different topic and explains why you should use the exercises, how they can help you, and what you can expect your progress to look and feel like.

Reformations Targeted by the Exercises in This Book

1. Always breathe at least 3 seconds in and 5 seconds out. Your breath should be a tiny but continuous sip of air that never pauses and always proceeds at the same rate.

2. Monitor your breathing carefully during conversations; don't let it become shallow.

3. Breathe through the nose as often as possible.

4. Minimize squinting, and raising your eyebrows.

5. Do not make your voice high pitched as an indication of affection or compromise.

6. Do not respond to provocation or threat with your face or with your breath.

7. Look above the horizon as much as possible.

8. After making eye contact, look at or above the eye line rather than below it.

9. The best posture for the neck is to look upwards while brining your chin to your chest.

10. Press your shoulders down and back, and flex your buttocks as often as possible.

11. Minimize replaying or imagining confrontational social scenaios.

12. Expect that the calmest version of you has what it takes to resolve any scenario.

13. Try being "dead calm," first by yourself and then with others.

14. Think of yourself as pure of heart, slow to anger, and not easily offended.

15. Make your posture and countenance ruthless, uncompromising, and unapologetic but temper this by making your personality humble, considerate, and affectionate.

Made in United States
Orlando, FL
04 October 2024

52356405R00080